DYING WAS EASY

LARRY J. KACHIK, MD

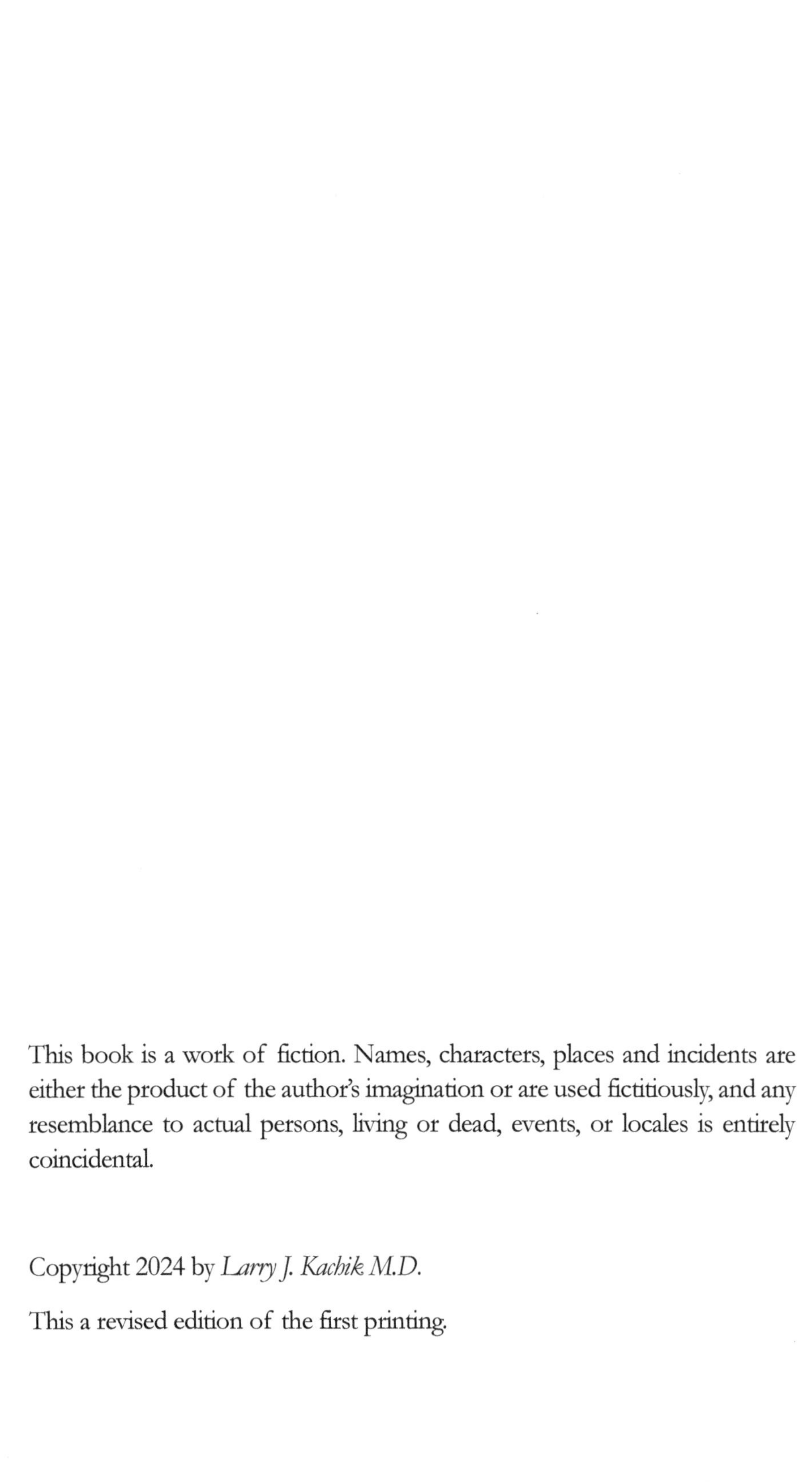

Table of Contents

AUTHOR'S NOTE

I don't follow rules well. In spite of the legalese on the previous page the character Tim Dempster was real. He was an incredible blacksmith. My horses won many races due in large part to his expertise. Tim passed away far too young. I honor his memory by including him. His name was used with the permission of his family. Miss you Timmy!

If I was terminal and wanted death to come soon, I would write non-fiction. I could research topics to try to put together a product that someone might want to read if they were stoned or otherwise impaired. That sounds to me like an assignment from high school or college. I avoided those as much as possible.

Fiction is different. I am free to exploit your imagination and mine. That is fun. This book is meant to be fun. Nothing in this book is meant to be real. So don't think any medical scenarios are completely accurate, and please don't do anything medical based upon what you read in this book. Likewise, the harness racing exploits are almost never consistent with current racing standards or rules. Any portrayal of legal proceedings is just that, a portrayal. I have made no attempt to achieve a factual display of jurisprudence. The language used may be a little salty to some. But if you have ever worked in an emergency department or hung out on the backside of a racetrack you will find it to be surprisingly familiar.

The inspiration for this book is my angel, Kathleen Marie Slifka Kachik. She was the person who had the most influence on me during my life. After ten years of dating, I wised up and married this amazing human being. She made every aspect of my life better. I was devastated when a cerebral hemorrhage called her to heaven at the tender age of fifty-four. During our incredible marriage she often commented that she wanted me to write a book. Most of that was prompted by her reading scathing emails that I had sent, that I had nicknamed "shitgrams." She was impressed with my ability to tell someone to "screw yourself" without saying it.

Well Kathleen, this is for you. I love you.

PROLOGUE

Interstate 28

Lakehurst, NJ

0915 December 5th, 2003

Fifteen feet behind them sat the motherload. The army grunts were clueless as to its existence. Their orders said that they were hauling twenty tons of tank parts to an army base in Nevada. That's the way the brass wanted it. Most movements of highly prized cargo utilized decoys. An up-and-coming officer crafted the brilliant idea of using the main caravan as a decoy. The prize was in this plain truck with no guards, and no fanfare. The theory was better than the outcome.

The driver lit another cigarette as his buddy slurped his half-cold, barely drinkable, gas station coffee. They entered the two-lane tunnel at the speed limit. About halfway through, their speed slowed when they saw flashing red lights near the exit. What they failed to notice was that after they, and the FedEx truck beside them, entered the tunnel, a police car stopped any more traffic from entering. The nearly empty tunnel smelled of exhaust fumes that quickly permeated the cab.

The army truck slowed, and stopped, as it neared the police car blocking the end of the tunnel. A badly overweight deputy slowly sauntered over to the driver's side of the vehicle. His taser, handcuffs, gun, and other policing paraphernalia swung gently from his rather large belt. The leather in his shoes and belt creaked as he walked.

"Accident?" asked the driver as he rolled down his window.

"No," said the deputy as he raised his arm and fired the revolver that he had concealed on his walk to the truck.

The first shot hit the driver in the temple, killing him immediately. The passenger dropped his coffee cup. Before he could do anything else, his head exploded from a well-placed second shot.

"Move your asses," yelled the deputy to the two men in the FedEx truck.

The driver deftly executed a three-point turn and backed up so his tailgate almost touched the tailgate of the army truck, which the deputy had lowered. It only took thirty minutes for the men to use hydraulic lifts to transfer the containers to the FedEx truck.

The deputy searched the pockets of the driver until he found the paper he needed. He pushed the bodies onto the floor on the passenger side and covered them with a tarp. Once the hood was opened, he easily found the tracking device. After attaching a small battery, he removed the device. Happy that the job was complete, he put the army truck back into gear and moved forward to the end of the tunnel. The flashing lights blocking the exit had vanished.

He reached for the radio mic as he exited the tunnel, but before he could talk, it squawked.

"Eagle One to Ground Hog One."

"This is Ground Hog One, go," the deputy calmly replied.

"Ground Hog One please give the password."

Fortunately, the deputy had gotten the information that the driver would be using a series of passwords based upon his location. The army driver had been kind enough to cross off the ones that had been used. The deputy just read off the next one on the list.

"Forty-six extra-large," he said slowly and deliberately into the mic.

"Roger that," replied Eagle One. "Why were you in that tunnel so long?"

"Accident, Eagle One, lucky we got through as quickly as we did."

"Roger, check in at your next milestone, Eagle One out."

The FedEx truck pulled off the road near the exit for the turnpike. It was a few minutes ahead of the empty army truck. The man in the passenger seat of the FedEx truck feverishly worked on his computer. He had a headset on with a mic. He put his finger to his lips to command the driver to remain silent. After ten minutes, when the appropriate number appeared on his screen, he keyed his mic.

"Gladstone County 911," he said very professionally.

"This is Captain Sam Killian of the US Army. I am tracking a convoy passing through your area and they were late with a check-in. Have there been any accidents?"

"Yes Captain, I can confirm that there was a two-vehicle accident at the westbound exit of the tunnel on Interstate 28 near mile marker 179. The call came in at 0423. The tunnel was briefly closed but has since reopened."

"Thank you, sir," replied Captain Killian.

Both occupants of the FedEx truck relaxed as the call ended. Had the captain checked with local EMS or police, as opposed to 911, he would have learned of the deception. But he hadn't. So, he didn't.

Back in the army truck, the deputy pushed the pedal to the floor. He had just stopped at a rest area and placed the tracking device on a truck that was headed in the correct direction. He knew the next check-in would be scheduled for anywhere from fifteen minutes to an hour from the last. He knew the password but not the location that would prompt him to call. But there would be no further calls. The tracking device would give the illusion that the truck was proceeding as planned until they didn't check in. The people monitoring the tracking device would not know for sure where the truck disappeared.

Around the next bend, he spied the turn he needed and took it. He proceeded for over ten miles down a gravel road and then he turned off into a pasture. He drove until he saw the ledge overlooking the river. He stopped the truck about a hundred yards short of the ledge and exited the driver's door. He removed a tire iron from the back of his seat and wedged it onto the gas pedal. He released the brake and jumped back as the truck lurched forward. It flew over the ledge at around 30 mph and disappeared into the deep river below. With any luck the army would not discover the truck missing until an hour or so from now. By then they would have around sixty miles of interstate to comb looking for clues. The chances of them finding the truck were slim to none.

The deputy sauntered back about fifty yards and recovered a motorcycle hidden behind a tree. He placed his helmet on and drove slowly retracing his route. There was no need to hurry now. The mission had been accomplished.

He arrived at the farm about thirty minutes after the men in the FedEx truck. They had pulled their truck into the large windowless storage shed. There, they were reunited with the two men and the police cars used in the tunnel. The four men began celebrating. Whiskey flasks were passed around. One of the men excused himself to whiz.

The deputy heard them singing, hollering, and carrying on. He waited for his brother to exit. He imagined the remaining men opening the cases of the pilfered cargo. All the while chugging whiskey and speculating as to how much they would each get. Unfortunately, some of the men had ties to the army. The deputy and his brother were almost certain the army guys would talk or somehow mess things up.

With a flip of a switch, the electronic locks on the garage door and the single-man door jumped into the locked position. The flip of a second switch started a large fan, which propelled deadly cyanide vapors into the shed. The party noise obscured the sound of the fan. No one noticed the smell of bitter almonds. It only took fifteen minutes for the process to be complete. The switch for the doors was flipped again, and the locks released. The large fan flow was reversed as the garage door opened.

The only noise now coming from the shed was from a radio playing rap music. The deputy and his brother clinked their beer cans together and scanned the room. The deputy shot his revolver at the radio and killed it. Three bodies laid in various contorted positions on the ground. All were lifeless, just as planned.

They needed to repaint both stolen trucks before they were delivered to a scrapyard that didn't ask too many questions. Then they had to dispose of the bodies. The only thing that remained unanswered was the question as to how they would celebrate their success.

CHAPTER 1

Emergency Department
Surfside Memorial Hospital
Atlantic City, NJ
2300 April 8th, 2022

"Hofucker, Hofucker, where are you?" I breathed into the tiny mic attached to my shirt.

"It's Hofecker, and I'm in room 15. Ron, are you sick? You don't sound like yourself."

"Tonight, it's Hofucker. You know that I have an e to u dyslexia."

"Shit ZZ, are you going to bust my balls all night about my name? Where the hell is Ron?"

"Hofucker, Ron and I switched shifts so I could get an early start on my vacation. Yes, of course, I am going to bust your balls all night. You are the resident, aren't you? Meet me in the hall outside of 15."

Another night, another full moon, and another resident physician with his head half stuck up his ass. With any luck, we may be able to extricate it before he graduates next year. Welcome to my life. I'm Zachary Zander. Most people call me ZZ, or asshole. I prefer ZZ. It's almost midnight April 9th, and it's a rocking night in the Surfside Memorial Hospital emergency department. Nothing good happens after midnight.

I'm your typical emergency physician, ridiculously handsome (if you ignore the horseshoe shaped scar on my face), intelligent, witty, and I am a smartass. I have nicknames for most people I like or hate. I try hard not to use their correct names. I have nicknames for people with inherently funny names regardless of my opinion of them, and I have a big Gadoonga. That's not the term I learned in anatomy, but I know you know what I mean. OK, so it's average size, but guess what? I get few complaints. Mr. Gadoonga, (I often refer to him as Mr. G), and I have had many exciting adventures. He seems to have a knack for getting into tight spots. But I'll save that for another time. We have work to do.

As one of the attending physicians in the ER tonight, I have two residents reporting to me. My third-year resident, Angela, is a dream. She's fast, but thorough. She gets along well with the patients, and the nurses just love her to death. Most people make this ER job much harder than it has to be. If you are nice to the patients, they will usually tell you what is the matter. If you are respected by the nurses, they will often give you the diagnosis, and they will kill themselves for you. Why do all the work if these people want to help? Angela is doing her last three months of training before she starts her life as an attending ER physician. Tonight, she will see more than her share of patients, bother me as little as possible, and maybe tell me a good, dirty joke. My kind of ER doctor.

On the other hand, there is Hofucker. Thomas Earhardt Hofecker III. Just the opposite of Angela. He is arrogant, lazy, and dimwitted. I suspect Daddy Hofucker II shipped plenty of greenbacks to the admissions office of the medical school (rhymes with Henn) that he attended. I am sure it took plenty more to keep him from getting booted out. He is a second-year resident, and in about twelve short weeks, he will be in his third year. He really isn't stupid, but he lacks common sense. ER is all about common sense. When I hear hoofbeats (I sweat bullets; more on that later), I look for horses. Internists look around for zebras. Neurosurgeons? Well, they are on a totally different wavelength. Hofucker's biggest weakness is that he doesn't know what he doesn't know. He thinks he is always right. Since I know he is mostly wrong, this is going to be a long shift.

Thank goodness for the wireless phone system we have. I can call him Hofucker all night, and only he and I can hear it. If I had to rely on an intercom, it would be Dr. Hofecker please call blah blah blah.

Hofucker stuck his head out of room 15 and made a circular motion with his finger on the side of his head.

"Are you trying to tell me this patient is nuts?" I asked.

"ZZ, you ARE sharp tonight!" he quipped. "Maybe you can help me, I need a few pearls of wisdom."

I put my arm on his shoulder and said, "Confucius says, 'Elevator smell different to short person.'"

Hofucker looked like he was going to cry. This dude needed to lighten up.

"What do you have?" I inquired.

"This guy is a whacko. His wife called the medics because he woke up screaming. He jumped out of bed and began rolling on the floor and banging his head on the wall. He claimed something was eating his brain. Cops had to taser him before the medics could get him on the stretcher. He is in four-point restraints, but still, as you can hear, he is carrying on something awful."

"What did your exam show, and what workup do you plan?"

"His blood sugar was 126. I think we need to sedate him with Ativan and Haldol and then CT him. We probably ought to get an ECG and labs to rule out cardiac damage from the taser and any metabolic problems. When all that comes back, we can clear him for admission to psychiatry."

"Hofucker, you scored points with the blood sugar. ANY altered level of consciousness requires a glucose assessment as soon as possible. I think I beat that into your head last month. I am glad you remembered to do one this time."

"Actually, the medics had done one on the way in."

See what I mean about this dude being a dim bulb? I just complimented him. He should have just accepted the praise. But then I should have known he would not remember. Thank God for good medics.

"What did your exam reveal?" I asked.

"Hard to do much of an exam with him in four- points. I thought I'd do a complete exam after we sedate and scan him."

That plan was lame for a second, and almost third, year resident. That's first year stuff. It costs nothing to examine the patient, and guess what? Every now and again, you make a diagnosis or at least narrow down your differential diagnosis. I swear people like Hofucker believe that they are "Bones" from *Star Trek*. They fantasize that if they wave a magic machine over their patients, the computer will give them the diagnosis. Time for a little teaching.

We entered the room together. The patient was about 30 years old with an athletic build. He was in his underwear and fixed to the stretcher with leather restraints. He had a few tasteful tattoos but no evidence of any trauma or bruising. Hofucker touched the patient's head, and all hell broke loose. The patient rocked back and forth on the stretcher until he almost turned it over. Hofucker called for security and told the nurse to get the Ativan and Haldol.

Security arrived and approached the bedside when I gave everyone the time-out signal. I made a T with my hands like they do in football. I then shooed everyone to the corner of the room and walked over to the gurney. I grabbed the patient's hand and shook it gently. I bent down to get near his face. Not too close, in case he was a biter. But I did risk a good hocker in the face if he was a spitter.

I said as calmly as possible. "Spencer, is that your name? Can I call you Spencer?"

No verbal response, but he shook his head.

"Spencer, I am sorry all of this happened to you. It's been a bad night. I know you were tasered, and I am sure you are tired of being in those restraints. I would like to help get you out of those as soon as it is safe for you and us. Please help me to help you."

He nodded.

"I need to ask you some questions and do a brief exam. But first, are you thirsty?"

See, I knew I had to win his cooperation, and to do so he needed to trust me. Offering a drink was a good first start.

He nodded in agreement.

"Bella, can you bring me a Coke?"

Bella was one of the RNs. Her real name was Sarah, but I always called her Sarahbellum. Like the part of the brain, the cerebellum. Then that got shortened to Bella. She was a good RN, and she was even better in the sack.

Bella peeled herself off the wall and returned with a Coke and a straw. Together, we sat Spencer up a little and he took a good pull of the Coke. He appeared to relax, then he started to scream and rock back and forth in the restraints.

"It's happening again!" he screamed. "It's eating my brain!"

Ignoring caution, I asked him which side.

He screamed, "Left!"

I grabbed an otoscope and looked in his left ear. Once I got past the earwax, I saw a nice light gray eardrum. Running laps on it was the diagnosis. A cockroach was doing donuts around the outside of his eardrum. I made Hofucker look and whispered something to Bella.

While we waited for Bella to return, I asked Hofucker how he would remove the offending creature. He pulled a pair of forceps from a locked cabinet and started walking toward the patient.

I almost shit. "Are you freaking crazy? With him thrashing around, you will end up burying those deep in his brain. You are going to pith the poor bastard. Guess again."

"OK." Hofucker put the forceps down and said, "We will paralyze him first and then remove the bug." He then listed off about six drugs he wanted to give as part of a rapid sequence induction of anesthesia and paralysis. He seemed so proud as he stood there with that dumb, but smug look on his face.

Just then, Bella returned with a single vial of medicine and drew up ten ccs into a syringe, and then discarded the needle.

"Score no points for that guess Hofucker. Watch and learn."

I took the syringe from Bella and squirted it in Spencer's ear. After an initial screaming fit, he seemed to calm down. I then took some saline and irrigated the ear. Out popped a stunned, but still alive, cockroach that fell to the floor. I peeked in Spencer's ear, and all was clear. We removed the restraints as Spencer looked over the side of the stretcher. Then he jumped up and landed foot first on the floor. His left foot crushed the offending insect with a crunch. Then he sat down and smiled.

Spencer then calmly relayed his story to us. "My place in Margate is being remodeled. My wife arranged for us to stay with her younger sister who is in college. I wanted to stay in a hotel, but with three dogs it is tough to find a place that will let you. So, we stayed with my sister-in-law. The place wasn't bad, but it's a rental for college kids, and not in a great neighborhood. No big deal. But I was none too happy when I saw a few cockroaches in a kitchen cupboard. In fact, before going to bed, I arranged for an exterminator to come today, even agreeing to pay triple time. My wife and I went to bed at 11 PM and soon thereafter, I felt something in my left ear. I could hear the damn thing crawling on my eardrum. I freaked out, and you know the rest of the story."

As it turns out Spencer was the CEO of an up-and-coming cybersecurity firm. I saw him on Fox Business a month or so after his ER visit. He later donated $1 million to the hospital for the care he received. That was nice for them, but he gave me squat. Just my luck. After all, I did save him from a malpracticing Hofucker.

Hofucker just stood there studying his navel and then he asked me what I flushed into Spencer's ear.

"Lidocaine," I said. "It incapacitates the bug so that it can be easily irrigated out. Let's see, I spent two dollars each for two syringes, six dollars for a bottle of lidocaine, and four dollars for some saline. A total of fourteen dollars. Your CT, paralysis, monitoring etcetera would have cost ten thousand dollars or more, and exposed the patient to unneeded risks. Here's where you blew it. You *ASSUMED* (I said with great emphasis) that Spencer was mentally ill, and you let that assumption cloud your judgment. You did not even attempt to get a history, and you did no exam. In just over a year, you may be alone some night in the ER, and hopefully, this experience will help you."

I was ready for a smart remark, but he simply bowed forward and said without sarcasm, "I bow to the master."

I then thanked the security staff and other nursing staff in the room. Before I left, I gave them a little advice about using four-point restraints.

"Use them with a hospital bed, not a standard ER gurney. When I was an intern, I saw a patient rock back and forth like Spencer was doing. Except that he flipped the cart over and broke his neck. He joined the paraplegic club, and the hospital lost a $20 million verdict. Food for thought."

Bella was obviously turned on by the whole event. She slid me a note as she left the room. All it said was: Breakfast at my place? Mr. Gadoonga stood up and applauded. I hope no one noticed as I waddled my way back to the nurse's station.

Over my earpiece came the piercing, high-pitched voice of Celeste, the unit secretary.

"Dr. Zander, unit 458 needs medical command."

CHAPTER 2

Emergency Department
Surfside Memorial Hospital
Atlantic City, NJ
0200 April 9th

On the way to the desk, my cell phone buzzed. I normally don't take personal calls at work, but it was from my mom. She never calls me.

"Mom, what is it? I really can't talk now."

"Zachary, it's about your father, he was badly hurt in an accident."

Before I could answer, the secretary screamed, "Dr. Zander, medic 458 is still waiting."

Sometimes I wanted to cold cock that bitch. The secretary, not my mom.

"OK, Celeste, don't get your panties in a wad. Mom, can I call you back in two minutes?"

"Sure Zachary."

I know the medics had to call me, but there are times that it just wasn't as important as what I was trying to do. ERs suck that way. Everything is a priority. I was really pissed when I found out that the reason my mother's important call was interrupted by the medics was because some druggie did not want to come to the hospital after an overdose. Before the medics could leave, the rule was that they had to call me. I really wanted to tell them to drop the asshole in the river, but that would take more time than I had. Instead, I told them that I felt great remorse that I would not be meeting the aforementioned drug addict. Believe it or not, I have a special place in my heart for addicts. Those that get help.

"Sorry Mom, please tell me about Carl." That's what I called my dad. We weren't very close.

"Zachary, you need to come home. Your dad was in an accident tonight. His truck hit a tree and he is in intensive care. He has tons of injuries, but they think he will survive. Ken Harrow was in the passenger seat, and he died." Mom lost it for a good minute. When she half composed herself, she said, "They say your father was drunk and he killed Kenny. Oh, Zach, what are we going to do?" The tears and sobs started anew.

"Mom this is my last shift here. After tonight, I have three weeks off. I get done at 7 AM and I will head home at that time. What hospital is Carl in? When I get a minute, I will try to get an update."

"OK Zach, you're a good son. I know you disagreed with what your father did to you, but please try to put it behind you. He, we all need your help. They took him to the hospital here in Krenshaw."

"I love you, Mom."

See what I mean about everything being a priority in the ER? I barely introduced myself to you and then we had to "bug out." You gotta admit that is now funny. Anyway, more background to get you up to speed.

Tonight, I will finish up a shift at Surfside Hospital, outside of Atlantic City. I do locum tenens emergency physician work. It sounds like something you might cough up or crap out, but it means I take temporary assignments in ERs around the country. I work when I feel like it, and I get to travel a lot.

As you heard, Carl is critically ill after a wreck. There was a time that that might have meant something to me. Now I feel bad for my mom, and my sister Stephanie, but I am ambivalent about Carl. I don't want to see him hurt, but I guess I am trying to tell you that I am not as upset as I ought to be.

Miraculously, it was a very slow night in the ED. Hofucker managed a couple of easy cases without killing anyone. Angela and the other attending offered to allow me to leave early, and I took them up on it. Mr. G was looking forward to breakfast with Bella, but we had to settle for a sausage breakfast muffin with egg. It was only an hour home. But after working most of the night shift, that's a haul. After wolfing down the sandwich, I planned to do a mega-caffeinated drink and a good cigar. That should get me there.

So, here's the scoop. Carl and Mom run a harness racing stable. They race some of their own horses and train others for paying clients. It's a tough business to make a living, but they did alright. I got fed and had decent clothes. We weren't rich, but we weren't on food stamps either.

We had a farm of about 200 acres and a very nice training track. Like all kids of farmers and horse trainers I did my share of work on the farm growing up. When I got old enough, I started to jog the horses. I eventually got to train them, and I really wanted to drive them in races. Carl was against it. Eventually, I wore him down and he relented.

Well, there are some things in life that you are naturally good at. With me, it's sex. Just kidding. I don't get many complaints, but I don't get much, so there are not many people to complain. But I will say that I was very comfortable behind a harness horse. As soon as I was old enough, I got my harness driver's license.

By the time I was nineteen, I was the leading driver at our local track, and by the time I finished college, I was one of the top drivers in the country. I made about $400,000 that year alone. When I got to medical school, I made a lot less because I could not take a lot of time off to drive. With classes and various clinical rotations, my time was limited. I wanted to be a Hall of Fame harness race driver. But I didn't want to be the doctor that killed a patient because he didn't know an axilla from an anus. So, my medical training took a priority.

I still managed to keep my name in circulation in the racing business. I picked up some live drives and decent bucks when I could arrange a day off. I had a Saturday off in August of my senior year and I picked up three drives at The Meadows racetrack outside of Pittsburgh. Two of them were good horses with decent chances to make money. One was a rat that had little chance to win, but the same trainer had all three. I had to take all three or take a powder.

The rat raced first and broke stride, finishing last. The second horse finished second and earned $30,000 purse money. I got 5%, and that worked out to $1500. Not bad for less than two minutes of work. I can resuscitate someone in the ER for thirty minutes and I am lucky to get paid about $200.

Anyway, the last of the three horses I was driving was the odds-on favorite to win $100,000 purse money. The $5,000 I would make when he won was dancing in my head as we left the gate. Within a few seconds that wasn't the only thing that was dancing in my head. The back right hoof of the four-horse caved in my face. The horse to the right of me broke stride out of the gate. He took a bad step and fell. My bike ran over his neck and that threw me off my bike and to the left. The four-horse reared up just as I was thrown onto the track. Number four came down to earth and planted his hoof in my face and the lights went out.

The next thing I knew it was ten days later. I woke up in the University of Pittsburgh Medical Center ICU on a ventilator. I had a serious head injury, and the trauma team hadn't given my parents much hope for me to live, let alone recover to a normal life. Being the cantankerous sonofabitch that I am, I decided to prove them wrong. Three months of rehab, and numerous scar revisions later, I was discharged.

I finished medical school and having been inspired by my experiences I chose a residency in emergency medicine. I did not choose plastic surgery because of the large facial scar that I inherited. I wasn't goofy (or smart) enough to be a neurosurgeon. I was very fortunate and very thankful, and by this time, very broke. All my harness racing money went to pay my medical bills and my medical school loans. OK, I should have had insurance, but I didn't. So, I move on.

Once I graduated from medical school, I wanted to start driving again. Unfortunately, Carl used his many contacts in the business to blackball me. Then, he had the nerve to call the insurance company that underwrote my disability insurance. Those dudes had to pay up big time in the event I became disabled and could not practice medicine. Nice protection. Well, their underwriters took a dim view of my harness driving career. They revised my policy and pretty much excluded any illnesses or injuries that could be related to racing.

Carl was very proud of having a son who was a doctor. When I got hurt, he decided that I would never sit behind a horse again. My racing career was over, and so was my relationship with Carl. We haven't talked since. I stayed close with my mom and my sister Stephanie who often visited me.

Carl and my mother's stable is called Fired Up Farms. It had initially been named FU Farms until the USTA (United States Trotting Association) made Carl change it. It was his private joke. He was under the radar until he named a filly FU Too. Someone in Columbus, Ohio, the home of the USTA, woke up. They banned the name, and he changed it to Fired Up Farms. All of the horses we bred or bought as yearlings contained the Fired Up moniker. It wasn't easy to make consistent money racing harness horses, but Mom and Carl did. It was even tougher when you had to help fund a school for special needs kids.

Mom called back with the added good news that in addition to being in critical condition, Carl would likely be arrested. He would be charged with homicide by vehicle while under the influence. He and Ken had stopped at The Daily Double. It was a semi-sleazy bar near the track that specialized in double-size drinks. Ken Harrow was a trainer who my father had been friends with for ages. Ken's wife had their first child that morning, and Carl wanted to buy him a drink. According to the police, they both were obviously drunk. They were playing pool in a back room. The bartender told them that he was shutting them off and would call them a cab. When the cab arrived, the pool room was empty, and Carl's truck was gone.

He smashed into a tree about a mile from the bar. Ken was riding with him and was ejected from the truck. Ken was pronounced dead at the scene with a broken neck. Carl was found alive in his truck. Somehow, he had enough sense to put his seatbelt on, even though he didn't have enough sense not to drive. He obviously neglected to ask Ken to put his seatbelt on. He was taken to the local hospital, Supreme Medical Center. He had a broken left arm, left leg, a collapsed left lung, numerous facial lacerations, and other minor injuries. My mom swore that although Carl would have one too many on frequent occasions, he never drove home. He either got a ride, took a cab, or she picked him up.

CHAPTER 3

Doctor's Parking Lot B
Supreme Medical Center
Krenshaw, NJ
0600 April 9

What arrogant asshole would name a hospital Supreme Medical Center? Were the Supremes in there? Probably some marketing dude who wanted to make people think the place was the supreme medical destination. In my experience, the more a hospital's name was made to sound like it was prestigious or provided excellent care, the worse the place was. One of the things Carl taught me prior to us severing our relationship was that if you were good enough, people would tell you. You wouldn't have to tell them.

It was obvious that the folks running this place never got that advice. The sign on top of the building proclaiming this to be the Supreme Medical Center was bigger than the scoreboard at Giants Stadium. This can't end well.

It didn't start well either. Being a doctor, I parked in the lot for doctors only. A portly security guard met me as I exited my vehicle.

"This lot is for physicians only," he said rather tersely.

"Well, that's nice, because I'm a physician. I am Dr. Zander, but you can call me ZZ." I held up my wallet, exposing a copy of my medical license, then I stuck out my hand.

He just shook his head, rocked back on his heels, and tried to look intimidating. Then he leaned forward and got in my face. His breath was horrible. Coffee, tobacco, and necrotic teeth make for a rather odoriferous combination.

"You might be a doctor, but you are not a doctor on this staff. I know all the doctors, and I don't know you. Now, move the truck."

"Your sign says, 'Parking for Physicians Only'. It doesn't specify that I have to be a member of your staff." After I made my point, I backed away to escape the fetid odor emanating from his oral cavity. I was now pissed, and damn close to barfing my breakfast. "Look pal," (I only say pal when I am pissed). "I am parking my truck here. I am here to visit a relative who is critically ill. There are plenty of spaces. I will move it as soon as I can, but for now, it stays here."

I stormed away as he babbled into his walkie-talkie. He would probably have it towed, but I'd deal with that later.

I had a rude awakening when I arrived at the entrance to Carl's ICU cubicle. I had taken care of many trauma victims, but it is more difficult to see a mangled body that belongs to someone to which you were related. Carl was covered with lacerations, bruises, bandages, and splints. He was on a ventilator and sedated. I was so disappointed in him. An accident I could understand. Killing your best friend because you drove drunk was unforgivable. After visiting him in ICU I went down to the ER. I was hoping to review his records.

The triage nurse looked like she was badly hungover and was battling a lethal case of PMS. She grunted to inquire as to the nature of my emergency. That was ER speak for "what the hell do you want?" I asked her to see if the ER director was in. Without looking up, she pointed me to a room across the hall. Beyond the restroom, which reeked of old urine that had missed the bowl, was a door with a small sign. It read Janet Dawson, MD, Director of Emergency Medicine. I knocked softly on the door.

"If you are selling, suing, or collecting, get the hell out of here." I heard clearly in a high-pitched voice.

"I am a fellow ER doc, and I am not selling, suing, or collecting."

"Well, enter then," the voice replied.

The office, although small, was much nicer than the waiting area. It smelled better than the odors wafting from the restroom next door, thanks to a candle on a conference table. The wall was covered with the usual documents verifying that Dr. Dawson had graduated from Penn State Hershey Medical School. She had completed her residency in emergency medicine at the University of Pittsburgh. She had passed her ER boards thereafter and was currently board certified in Emergency Medicine. Ok, she had the creds.

"What is your name again?" she asked. She, too, looked irritated. It made me wonder. Was she related to the security guard or the triage nurse? Is everyone in this whole place pissed off all day, every day?

"I am Zachary Zander. I am an ER physician, and I was hoping to see Carl Zander's chart. He is my father." I almost choked on that last sentence. I hated to admit he was my father, but I thought my relationship, strained as it may be, might help me get access to the chart. "He was severely injured in an accident last night."

The bitch just stared at me. Was it the scar on my face? Did I have a booger hanging from my nose? Sausage stuck in my teeth.

So, I glared back at her. She was about thirty-five going on fifty. She might have been a babe once, but the crow's feet and extra heft she was carrying, about twenty pounds, made her look quite plain. That was being generous. What once might have been a vivacious figure was accented by two floppy breasts that couldn't pass the pencil test. (Place a pencil under the breast, if the pencil falls out the breast is firm. That is good. If it gets stuck under the breast, that is bad.) She also had a severe case of MOA. Mushed Out Ass syndrome. Common malady where a once round and attractive butt expands its borders. MOA is characterized by ill-defined ass-leg boundaries. You can't tell where the ass stops, and the leg begins.

Silently I told Mr. Gadoonga, "Cut that shit out. We aren't here in pursuit of breakfast for you." In fact, we had just passed up a great invitation. No wonder he was irritated and so critical.

I cleared my throat and said, "I am sorry to bother you, but I am just trying to get a handle on what happened with my father."

"As an ER physician, you would know I can't help you get the records. You will need to follow the procedure in medical records to see them."

"I imagine that will take about two weeks, am I right?" I asked nervously. She was definitely staring at my face.

"Were you once a harness race driver?"

"Yes, I was. I may be going back to it, why do you ask?"

"During my residency at Pitt, I was on a trauma call for a harness race driver who had his face stepped on at The Meadows racetrack. Was that you?"

"Ah, that's why you are fixated on the scar! That was me."

"Wild case. Sorry about the scar, but you have no idea how bad that wound looked. That was peanuts compared to the head injury. You are lucky to be alive."

"Yeah, I am. I have you and the trauma team at Pitt to thank. The scar doesn't bother me. In fact, it gives me class." I laughed to be kind, but of course, it bothered me.

She held out her hand. "Janet, Janet Dawson. Zach, is it"?

"ZZ," I told her.

In the next five minutes, she transformed from a pudgy, homely, bitchy doctor to a colleague who was happy to see that I was alive and well. She wasn't beautiful, but she was gracious and kind. Mr. G had it all wrong this time.

After catching up and comparing careers, we concluded that ERs everywhere were very similar. After a phone call, a printed copy of Carl's record magically appeared on her desk. Janet coincidently had to go to the restroom. She didn't hand me the chart, but when she left me alone with it, I got the signal. She wanted me to see it. But she needed plausible deniability that I had purloined it, as opposed to her giving it to me. Hence the sudden need for her to take a squirt.

The records were devastating to read. In addition to all the injuries and scans, I saw that his blood alcohol was 0.260. The legal limit was 0.08. Wow, he was wasted. I was so embarrassed. Carl was a drunk piece of shit… Can't get much lower than that. I could barely look Dr. Dawson in the eye when she came back.

"I feel badly for you," she said. "No one likes to see their parent in a bad light. Today, you got to see him near death and now you know why. That has to hurt. I'm so sorry."

"The truth can be very painful. I appreciate your help and your kind words. I've got a lot of stuff to sort out. My father is very likely to be incarcerated, my mother can't run our business alone. Lots of things to digest."

"I hate to sound insensitive, but if you plan to come back to the area, I may have a job for you. Pending, of course, on a thorough background check and references. Keep me in mind," Dr. Dawson added as she pressed her card into my hand.

CHAPTER 4

Fired Up Farms
Krenshaw, NJ
0900 April 22

Carl received excellent care. He went from the hospital to an inpatient rehab facility. I couldn't bring myself to visit him in the hospital or rehab. I just didn't want to see him. Mom visited him daily. I kept myself busy helping with the horses and the farm. I was utterly disgusted with the condition of the place.

I hadn't been home for three years. The farm I remembered was pristine. Not a blade of grass out of place. It had an incredible training track that was immaculately maintained. The farmhouse was equally impressive. The barn was a sight to see. Perfectly appointed and painted. Landscaped with meticulously tended grass, shrubs, and hundreds of annual flowers. Mom had selected them appropriately so that something was blooming from April through October.

What I saw when I got home made me sick. The horses were well-fed, and the barn interior was perfect. I knew my mom and Carl would starve themselves to death before any of the horses would receive less than stellar care. But other than the horse's living quarters, the place looked like shit. The grass along the outside of the barn hadn't been cut in quite a while. No wonder. The riding lawnmower and the push mower would not start. The tractor started but coughed and smoked so much that I shut it down for fear of a fire.

There were no annuals except for a few volunteers that were remnants from years gone by. They were hard to see through the tall weeds that engulfed them. The fencing was badly in need of a coat of paint. The training track had only been maintained at the rail. Eighty percent of it was rutted and unusable. The farmhouse was even worse. The screen door on the front entrance hung from one hinge. A broken window had been boarded up instead of repaired. Pieces of aluminum siding were missing in action. A tarp covered a section of the roof that must have leaked. I was so distracted as I walked in that I almost tripped on a loose board on the front steps. Why was the place so run down?

Mom only cried when I asked her. She told me to ask Carl. She begged me to visit him. I just couldn't bring myself to do it. I was still pissed and now I was ashamed that he murdered his friend while driving drunk. How could I possibly give a shit about anything he had to say?

While he recovered, I busied myself with resuscitating the home and farm I grew up in. After three weeks and $25,000 out of my pocket, I had most of the glaring deficiencies corrected. The roof was fixed. The window was repaired. The porch and front entrance were made safe.

The grass was cut after all tractors and mowers were restored to a functional status. Annuals were planted as weeds were culled. I spent the last three days working on the training track. I logged twenty hours in the tractor furrowing and smoothing it back into condition. I used that quiet time to try to put things in perspective.

Dad killed his best friend while driving drunk. Our farm and house were in complete disarray. My mother looked like a zombie. My sister Stephanie was a zombie.

Stephanie is my adopted sister. They say she has some type of autism but don't tell her that. She might hurt you. I love Stephanie and she loves me. She is the sweetest person. But with her condition, there is sometimes a wall between her and the rest of the world. She is highly intelligent, but oftentimes, she just can't, or won't, communicate. You never know if she will speak or not. If she does talk, every other word is often vulgar. But vulgar is at least talking, and I'll take that. She is petite but wiry. All of 5 feet 4 inches and weighing in at 104 pounds with flowing curly blonde hair. Although she is twenty years old, she could pass for fifteen.

My parents adopted her when she was twelve. Her father, Stan, was a harness trainer and driver, and a good friend of Carl. Stan died in a horrible racing accident when Stephanie was seven. Apparently, it isn't safe to be a harness racing buddy of Carl. When Stan was killed, Stephanie's biological mother totally lost it. She found solace by killing off a fifth a vodka a day. That pissed off her liver and it quit. She cashed her chips when Stephanie was nine. Stephanie bounced from institution to institution for the next three years. She had never spoken. She had very poor balance and coordination. She needed tons of therapy that she never received. Mom and Carl visited her regularly, but she was unable to acknowledge their presence. That little girl's life only turned around thanks to Justin McGregor and Always Hope.

Justin was Carl's principal owner. He was infatuated with harness racing. Justin was a typical entrepreneur. He started ten businesses, most of which failed. The ones that didn't did exceptionally well. He married his childhood sweetheart, Hope. Unfortunately, Hope succumbed to a very aggressive breast cancer at the age of thirty-five. Justin was devastated but he was one tough dude. A trivial matter like death was not going to separate him from his true love.

A few months later, Carl found a trotting filly at a sale that he liked. Mom loved her pedigree for future breeding. On their urging, Justin bought her and named her Always Hope.

She was a big mare, and she lived up to her name on the racetrack. If she was on the track, there was always hope that she could win. She won on the front end, and she came from behind to win. She found many paths to victory, and she took them often. I drove her until my accident, and she was pure joy. She let you drive her to a certain point. If she thought you were screwing up, she made her own move, and you were just a passenger. She won 42 races over three years and brought in purses of $2,000,000.

As it turns out, Justin was at the farm one day that Stephanie visited. Justin was in the paddock giving Always Hope a peppermint candy. They were her favorite treat. Mom and Carl brought Stephanie out. They practically had to carry her. Carl set her down near the fence to the paddock and a miracle happened.

Stephanie ran, more like stumbled, between the fencing and waddled over to Always Hope. Stephanie staggered up to the big mare and rubbed her chest. Always Hope nudged Stephanie with her chin.

Then Stephanie spoke. "Nice fucking horse, nice fucking horse."

Those were the first words anyone ever heard her speak. Her time in institutions obviously taught her the F-bomb. F-bomb or not, Mom and Carl were ecstatic. Justin broke down and cried. He knew his departed wife's work when he saw it and heard it. He knew what he had to do, and Justin knew how to turn dreams into reality.

My parents adopted Stephanie and brought her home to the farm. Justin demanded to pay for therapists to come to the farm to work with her. He was not someone who understood the word no. Within a few days of her adoption, she was evaluated and had a treatment plan created by psychiatrists, physical therapists, occupational therapists, and speech therapists. Over the next few years, Stephanie made amazing progress. Most of her days were spent with the horses. She and her therapists worked their therapy around the horses. Whether it was walking them, grooming them, or just cleaning out stalls, every task had a therapeutic end game. It was obvious to all that she had a special bond with her equine friends. The therapists capitalized on that. Stephanie and the horses had their own form of communication.

Her incredible progress prompted Justin to envision The Always Hope School. It was one of the better things that Carl assisted in bringing to life before he started to make license plates. It was a school for special needs kids that just weren't cutting it anyplace else. After Justin saw the gains that Stephanie had made, he encouraged friends and employees to bring their kids with special needs to the farm. He saw to it that they all got an in-depth evaluation and a treatment plan.

It was around this time that one of Justin's businesses took off. He was rich beyond even his wildest dreams. And trust me, this guy was a dreamer. He asked my mom and Carl's permission to build The Always Hope School on our farm. His dream was to build a model to manage these kids that could be replicated throughout the country. With his donation of $10,000,000, his dream became a reality. He then set up an endowment of $100,000,000 to fund the school in perpetuity. Justin did things in a big way.

Unfortunately, perpetuity was about as short-lived as Justin McGregor. Within a month of signing the papers, he developed a fever and severe headache. He was in Boston and ended up at Brigham. That's a fancy smansy Harvard Medical School teaching hospital. A snooty place, but the care was exceptional. Mom asked me to fly up to see him, but Justin never knew I was there. He was comatose, and on a vent. He had an amebic brain infection and was dead in 48 hours. Apparently, a few days before, he had been swimming in a lake near the farm.

Shortly after that, I had my accident. It was a long recovery. When I completed rehab, I worked hard at hating Carl. I had frequent visits from Stephanie and Mom when I was back in Jersey between locum ER assignments, but I never went back to the farm until a few weeks ago.

At dinner that night, Mom could only say "thanks." I knew she was very happy with what I had accomplished, but her emotional fuel gauge was on empty. She was a shell of the "tough as nails" woman that had raised me. That's why it was so difficult to refuse her when she asked me to pick up Carl tomorrow. I tried as hard as I could to say no. Her brown, bloodshot eyes simply would not permit it.

CHAPTER 5

New Vista Rehabilitation Hospital
New Vista, NJ
0900 May 6

I arrived in his room with my arms full of things for him. My mom had packed clothes and shoes. She got up early and made chocolate chip cookies. The only thing I had to offer him was disdain. I set the stuff down and settled into a chair facing him. His nurse had told us that we were only waiting for the doctor to come to officially discharge him. There was silence in the room when she left. After a few long minutes, Carl spoke.

"Zach, I know you have been upset with me for pushing you out of harness racing. You were one of the best. But I just couldn't stand the thought of you having another accident. You are too good of a doctor and a person to lose like that."

"Well Carl, I really wish you would have let me make that decision. Instead, you used your connections to blackball me out of the business. Calling the insurance company was the last straw. I made a vow to be pissed at you forever. So far, I have kept the vow."

"Zach, you know what I did was wrong, killing Ken and all." He fought back some tears and then continued. "I know that you have lined up an excellent defense attorney that I can't afford, and that I don't need."

"Carl, if you need anything now, you need the best attorney. You are looking at ten to twenty years in prison. You might get out in five to ten, but every year makes a difference."

"I know what you are saying, but I know I am guilty. I don't want any defense. I just want to face the judge and accept my sentence like the man I hope to become. I used to think I was a good man, but good men don't kill their best friend on the day his first son was born." He choked up a little and continued. "Zach, I have to ask you to do something I never thought I would. I need you to run the farm and the racing operation. I'd prefer you not drivebut I will leave that up to you. Your mother will need a lot of help. I know I have no right to ask. I also know you have every right to walk out of here and go on with your life. But I wish you wouldn't."

I needed a lot more information before I could give him an answer.

"Carl, what the hell is going on? When I last was home the school was going big guns, Fired Up Farms was the number one stable in harness racing, and the farm and house were pristine. I haven't been to the school, but it looks ok from the outside. The stable barely wins enough to feed the horses. The farm and house are (were) shitholes."

"Your mother told me that you fixed up a lot of things. Thank you. I will repay you, someday." Carl said with great remorse.

"I don't care if you repay me, but you do owe me some answers."

Our discussion was interrupted by the doctor's arrival. After a brief exam, Carl was discharged. We packed up his things, and they pushed him out to the car in his new wheelchair.

On the way home, Carl told me the story. I was right. Three years ago, things were going great. Then Justin McGregor died. Carl was quick to point out that initially, he thought Justin's death would have little effect on the school and stable. After all, the school had no mortgage and was fully funded by a $100 million dollar endowment.

He knew the stable would be impacted. Not too much initially because all of Justin's horses were to be raced under his estate with any profits to go to the school. Carl didn't lose any of the horses, but he could not purchase any new ones for Justin's estate. But as a top trainer he was sure he could attract more owners.

"That's about the time that things went to hell." Carl went on to relay how, almost overnight, things changed at the track. His horses were going as fast as ever, but they were consistently getting beat. He fell from the top stable in the state to one that barely eked out an existence.

"Why???" I thought he might have an idea.

"Damn if I know for sure. Supreme Stables lured Carlton Hennessey here and instantly, they took total control. He had been a successful trainer in

Canada but nowhere near as successful as he became here. We found ourselves racing for second and third place checks most nights, and that didn't do much for the bank balance. Slowly but surely, your mother and I dipped into savings and cashed in our retirement accounts. That bought us some time until we were blindsided by another shitstorm. Justin had sold most of his last business to a group of venture capitalists. That's what funded the endowment for the school. Justin's will was ironclad. However, the venture capitalists wanted their $100 million back. The slimy bastards claimed that Justin had made them promises."

"What kind of promises?"

"They claimed that he promised to give them back their money if he wasn't able to advise them how to run the business. It took a year but eventually a judge ruled in their favor. They got $85 million from the endowment. Their snake attorneys were better than ours. I guess you never heard about this or saw the ad?"

"I did my best to avoid reading anything about harness racing or the school. What was the ad about?"

Carl continued. "Your mother was so mad when the last appeal was lost that she got the name of every investor who had sued. She bought a full-page ad in the *NY Times* that included a picture of Always Hope being groomed by two of our special children. The caption read, 'Do you know any of these investors?' Then it listed all of them, including their name, addresses, and, when available, phone numbers. It went on to say 'These ruthless individuals obtained $85,000,000 intended to benefit the care and education of special needs children. Ask them about it!'"

I had to grin. Mom was like a volcano, quiet until she wasn't. She had doxed the bastards.

Carl also had a smile on his face as he completed the story. "From what I heard; her project was a success. As long as six months later, the investors were still getting nasty calls and letters. One bitter soul tossed a bag of horseshit on an investor's Mercedes. Nah, it wasn't mom. Honest. But I don't know where Stephanie was at the time."

Carl's smile was quite short-lived as he recalled the events of the last year. "After the haircut the endowment took, it could not fund the school. We thought we could get by for five years by using the principal. We hoped to find permanent funding before it ran out. The kids in the school were making amazing progress. We thought if we had a track record, we could attract the cash to fund the endowment again."

I was shocked to hear the story. "I had no idea; why didn't you or Mom tell me? I saw her and Stephanie often, and no one said a word."

Carl bowed his head. "I wouldn't let them. I knew I had wrongly interfered in your life once. I had no right to do it again. Things were ok until the final shoe dropped. I think your mother's ad really pissed some people off. The venture capitalists came back for the final $15 million. They managed to freeze any use of the principal until the case was heard the next year. So, we only had the interest on the $15 million to fund the school. We considered cutting the number of kids in the school, but each case was so special that we couldn't do that. So, we mortgaged and borrowed and cobbled together short-term funding. The therapists at the school took a voluntary thirty percent pay cut to help. They are great people. They believe in us and the school, and most importantly, the kids. Our attorneys feel that we can prevail in the suit next year. But Zach, the vultures are circling. We are out of cash and running out of time. And instead of helping, I am going to prison."

I then saw something I never saw before and hope to never see again. My dad bawled his eyes out. He struggled to get control as we pulled into the driveway.

"Zach, you are a good son. Please help us. Do it for your mother and sister and those great kids. I don't deserve your help or respect. Although someday I might."

When we got home, I wheeled him into the house. Mom ran over and gave us both vigorous hugs. Her eyes were still bloodshot from way too many tears.

"Where's Stephanie?" whispered Carl.

"In her room, she's regressed. She won't eat. She's lost ten pounds that she could ill afford to lose." Mom got the words out between sobs.

When I got to her room, I found her sitting in a chair facing the corner of the room like a child being punished. She was rocking back and forth. She did not acknowledge my presence. I walked over and kissed her on the forehead. She never looked up, never blinked, and never stopped rocking.

"Stephanie, Dad is here. You want to go see him?" It almost made me choke to call him "Dad", but I did it for her. I knew that communication with her had to be clear and precise.

She did not respond.

"Stephanie, I know this is difficult for you. Dad will being going away for quite a while, and I know he wants to see you."

No response.

I then tried to lift her from the chair. Out of nowhere she hit me with a right hook that I swore came from Mike Tyson. My eyes watered and I nearly passed out. I don't think she broke my jaw, but she could have.

She was still rocking but now chanting "motherfucker, motherfucker, motherfucker" on and on and on.

Best words I could ever hear. When she went into a trance, she usually came out of it chanting. Maybe we could move on. I just stood there and watched for a few minutes. Then she stood up and threw her arms around me. She was still chanting but I was getting hugged instead of mugged.

CHAPTER 6

Municipal Courthouse

Krenshaw, NJ

1000 May 21

Carl pleaded guilty to homicide by vehicle while under the influence. He said he could not remember anything other than arriving at the bar. He accepted that he had done it and didn't fight the charges. He did allow our personal attorney to represent him. He got a sentence of seven years, but he could be out in three with good behavior. The judge was moved by Carl's admission of guilt and willingness to accept the consequences of his actions.

Mom swore on a stack of Bibles that she never knew him to drive after taking even one drink. But the evidence showed that he had driven, and the result was a dead friend. He took up residence at the state penitentiary in Driftwood.

Prior to his incarceration I got my friend PC to do a thorough audit. His name is Johnson Stevens. PC is short for "pisscatcher". During college PC had a part-time job at the track collecting urine samples after races. He got them from the horses, not pissed off patrons. Once he graduated and obtained his CPA, he still worked part-time at the track. He liked betting and he got a lot of inside tips. Although he was up to his ears in work, he dropped it all when I called. He had a preliminary report in just three days, and it was a nightmare.

The biggest problems were the expenses for the school. The best he could figure is that the school owed about $1,000,000 in back taxes and about $5,000,000 more in short, and longer-term loans. The true cash burn rate was about $400,000 a month. PC wanted us to close the school, sell the farm, equipment, and all the horses. If we did that, we could walk away clean.

Mom would not hear of it. Her and Carl had turned down numerous offers over the past year. She wasn't selling the farm, and although she was willing to sell a few of the horses, she would never sell Always Hope. She would never close the school, period, end of story. Stephanie and The Awesome Army (that's what Stephanie called the kids in the school) were flourishing wildly with therapy and education. Mom even thought that we could publish our success and possibly encourage other schools to form. Hope and Justin McGregor's dreams were still very much alive in my mom! On the verge of financial ruin, husband in the hoosegow, and she was still ready to fight.

By now, Stephanie was twenty. She had turned into a beautiful young lady. Her therapy had helped her strength and balance. She regularly jogged even the toughest of the racehorses and she did it with ease. Her language skills were improved but were not optimal. She might have Tourette's in addition to autism, was all the professionals could guess. You never knew what Stephanie would say.

PC and I met with the creditors. They wanted everything now, and I offered nothing. It was immediately apparent that the farm was the asset that was the center of attention. Always Hope was also of considerable interest. After a few hours of diddling around, the main creditor offered to forgive all past due payments in return for immediately turning over the farm to them, plus Always Hope. Mom could keep the other horses. It was the deal of the century.

Always Hope was in foal to Dahanana. He was the harness horse of the year two years ago. I had Always Hope and her soon to be foal's value privately appraised at $1,500,000. It wasn't what I wanted to do, but I had to ask Mom to go along. I thought she would get mad, or cry, or cry madly. She did nothing.

She got up and walked out to the barn and entered Always Hope's stall. She put a halter on her head and led her out into the sunshine. She walked her over to me and handed me the rope.

"Do what you think is right," she said.

She petted her as I stood there looking into these big brown eyes attached to this beautiful animal. I led her back into her stall and called the creditor's attorney.

"No deal, pal."

"Dr. Zander, we are giving you a chance to walk away from this. You have a promising medical career, and your family can go back to racing but without the farm and the horse."

"You cocksucker, you know that my parents have the school to worry about. They can't just walk away."

"Listen to me, you stupid ass ER doctor. Isn't that where doctors go to work who can't practice real medicine?"

I was synthesizing my rebuttal when he continued.

"The gloves are off, you asshole. I am telling you that there are a number of creditors that will still end up losing millions, even with this deal. I can honestly tell you that they have no interest in racing or breeding Always Hope. They plan to turn her into dog food, and they plan to send your mom the tape of the butchering. That *NY Times* ad really set them off."

"Hey, big shit barrister. Check this out. I will have $100,000 by the end of the week. I will pay $6000 a week until The Miracle Mile concludes on August 23. At that time, I will either have $6,000,000 more for you, or you get title to everything, including Always Hope."

"Unacceptable Zander, we have waited far too long for our money. We are going to close you out."

"Don't think so, moron. You and I both know that this can be dragged out. I got word to the judge that I intend to make good on our settlement. You damn well know he won't close us out if we can still pay, even if it is slowly. Checkmate. Eat shit and die." I hung up.

I quit my locum work. Janet Dawson still needed a physician. I was hired at Supreme Medical. In order to work the horses in the morning and race in the evenings, I had to take a full-time position as the physician on the 12 AM to 7 AM shift. I got the word out at the track that I was back and ready to race. Having been out of the sport for years would not encourage a lot of trainers to use me. I would have to impress them while mostly driving our horses. If I won, I would get more drives; if not, I would have to find much more money.

CHAPTER 7

Route 17 N

Krenshaw, NJ

2340 June 2

On my drive to the hospital for my first shift, I pondered what it would be like to sit behind a horse in a real race. I couldn't tell anyone, and didn't really want to admit it to myself, but I was terrified. I still had flashbacks from the start of the wreck I had been in. I don't remember much but what I did was bad. I was able to watch the tape of the race many times. Every day when shaving, I look at the horrible scar on my face. It's hard to look pretty after a horse stomps on your face. Tomorrow night, I will get to see if I can drive a horse competitively again.

I arrived at the ER at 2355. Not knowing where the employee entrance was, I walked into the main entrance to the emergency department. That was my first mistake. The sights and sounds of that waiting room were stunning. A guy with no shirt, shoes, or pants was standing in the corner, pissing on the Coke machine. Babies were crying and people were vomiting in trash cans. The floor was accented with puddles of blood that gushed from wounds that should have been closed hours ago. I worked my way to the triage desk as patients reached out to try to get my attention. I felt like Jesus walking through a leper colony. I wanted to help them, but I had to get into the ER to do it best. The only thing between me and the ER was one door and a Jenny.

The door was a standard door, but it was locked. I had no key or entry code. The Jenny was a charge nurse about 5 '11 who weighed about 125 pounds soaking wet. She was dry now and appeared to be pissed off about something. There had to be something in the air, everyone here was always pissed. She had auburn hair cut far too short, and despite some very unflattering scrubs, she was hot. Mr. G wondered what it would be like to pin those long legs behind her ears. That peaceful thought was interrupted by a screech.

"Where the hell have you been?" screamed Jenny as she opened the door.

"Huh, I am Doctor Zander, and this is my first shift," I replied meekly.

"No shit, Sherlock," retorted Jennie. "We have been calling you for two hours. You are required to be available to start your shift up to two hours early depending on demand, and tonight we demanded. I hope you don't plan on pulling this crap too often," said Jenny with her hands on hips.

My first instinct was to smack her and go home. Then my mom would lose the school and farm, and I probably would get sued.

I bit my tongue and said, "Sorry, no one had told me that."

Jenny wrinkled up her forehead, got a little smile on her face and offered me her hand.

"Jenny Rich, charge nurse. This is my shift, and this is my passion. I have no life outside of here and today I also have a damn migraine. So-sorry. Welcome to Supreme Medical. We are about six hours behind but today is your lucky day. I am going to attach myself to your skinny ass so we can move the meat and get caught up. I might even want to get to know more about you later if you impress me. Do you want to get in the AON contest?"

"Sure, how much?" I asked.

"$3, winner takes all. Contest closes at 6 AM and we vote at 0630."

I was somewhat surprised to hear that the AON contest was widespread. I had played before in Atlantic City, but being a gambling town, I figured it was a local custom. At least I understood the rules.

AON stood for "asshole of the night." The staff that elected to play (they all did) selected a contestant from the players of the night. The players included patients and relatives, and friends of patients. All participants voted at 0630, and the holder of the winning asshole got the entire purse. It was a tough competition. Assholes in the ER on the night shift were a dime a dozen. But which asshole would be the best (or worst)? You only got one selection and the first to make it got the person. So, you have to be quick. If you picked too soon you might miss the flamer to arrive later. If you waited, you might lose to a quiet night or a night full of legitimately sick people. Jenny informed me that the winnings were customarily spent to buy eye-openers at the Daily Double. The night shift staff often ended up there after work, and yes, that was the same bar Carl was in.

Some people thought it was crass for us to "make fun of patients." For the most part, we didn't, but some of these people were true assholes. ER personnel are very down to earth. They call balls and strikes. In addition to that, they work under incredible pressure. Say you start your shift with a very sick child who may die, or a rape, or a severely wounded domestic violence patient. How do you finish the rest of your shift? You have to leave it on the field and move on. Playing AON was one way to do that. If you don't understand, don't ever think about working in an ER.

"I am in." I threw three dollars at Jenny, set down my briefcase and got to work.

I scanned the computer board displaying the information we had on patients. I quickly determined that there were twenty-three patients in rooms or the waiting room waiting to be seen. I clicked on the chart of the next to be treated and low and behold, I may have the winner already. Hating nights or not I loved the ER, and I settled in to show Jenny and the troops that I was a player. I also bet my $3 on my first patient. I couldn't believe that no one had snatched him up.

"Don't let me down dude."

His emergency was "carrot stuck up ass." You have got to love it. Jenny had a half smile on her face. I wondered whether this was some kind of joke, but I had to play it out. We walked in silence back to the room, knocked on the door, and went in. A hairy-chested fifty-something guy with tons of ink looked up from the exam table.

"Don't even fucking ask," he said as I was about to inquire about the misplaced vegetable.

I just looked at him as I silently thought. Of course, this is a common occurrence. You were jumping into the shower when your phone that you had left in the kitchen rang. You ran back to the kitchen to answer the phone and slipped. You tried to steady yourself by grabbing the counter but all you did was push a carrot off the counter. The carrot fell point up into the dog's water bowl. As you fell, the carrot went right up your ass. Yep, happens all the time.

I was thinking it but there were times that you didn't need to ask how something occurred. With Jenny's help, we got him undressed and I did a rectal exam. I could feel something at the end of my finger, but this thing was in deep. Jenny recommended that I call a surgeon. "No one can get those out," she said. I was thinking that this community abuses their vegetables a little too much for her to know this, but I asked her to get me a sigmoidoscope.

"Look here doc, I have seen this movie three or four times. The doctors get the scope and piddle around for an hour or so, and they can never get the thing out. Dildos, carrots, bananas, it all ends the same. Eventually they call a surgeon, who takes the patient to the operating room after we wasted a good hour. Do me a favor and consult the surgeon."

"Yo Jenny, you are going to have to learn something about me. I am one cocky and stubborn SOB. I plan to have this carrot ready for your dinner tonight."

The scope came and within a few minutes, the base of the carrot was staring at me through the scope. I grabbed the carrot with some forceps and tried to pull, no go. I readjusted and pulled again. This time, I got a bite-size piece of carrot, but the rest was still in a dark place. Then I remembered an article I read in a throwaway journal. The problem was that the colon was squeezing the carrot. As I pulled the carrot it actually increased the suction on the carrot.

I asked for a red rubber catheter and wedged that between the carrot and the descending colon. I added a dollop of KY jelly and gently pulled the carrot out. Jenny was amazed. I put the carrot in the trash. Jenny went to the desk and the patient went to the restroom to get dressed. I pulled the carrot back out and snapped a picture showing the thick end of the carrot with a small piece missing. Revenge is a dish best served with a carrot.

The next three patients were all drunk. I could never figure out why ER docs get so pissed at drunks when most ER docs drink like fish when they can. I think they are just jealous that when they are on duty the patients can drink and they can't. I repaired two lacerations, which were pretty easy work, and then I hit the brick wall. Chief complaint, "severe vaginal odor." Great, some people that stink don't know that they do. When they know there is something foul you better be prepared. Most ER personnel are experts at breathing through their mouths to avoid pungent odors. On rare occasions when that didn't work, I tried an old trick from the stable. I'd put Vick's in my nose. Sometimes, at the track or barn, our stallions would get all bent out of shape if they smelled a filly or mare in heat. A dab of Vick's in their nose sometimes got their thoughts back on their business.

I elected to try it without the Vicks, a decision that I would soon regret. As we arrived in the room, we encountered a twenty-three-year-old female who could barely make eye contact with us. What eyes we saw were red. Via badly slurred speech, she stated that three days ago, she noticed a vaginal odor which had gotten worse. She had a small amount of discharge. The nose breathing was working quite well as we set her up for a pelvic exam. At first, I found nothing. Then I repositioned the speculum under her cervix so I could see the space between her cervix and the posterior vagina. There it was…a dead gray mouse! Was there a deceased rodent in her vagina?

Not really. It wasn't a mouse, but it looked like one. It was a tampon that had become lodged in that space. I got my forceps and removed it without incident. Then it started. Once that tampon hit the air the most disgusting smell imaginable immediately filled the room. It was a combination of rancid meat and vomit. Pretty typical of a severe overgrowth of anaerobic organisms. Those are the ones that grow best in an environment without oxygen. There wasn't much oxygen where I found it. Despite bagging up the odoriferous object and cleaning the room it was over two hours until we could use that room again.

"Jenny, did you step on that tampon?"

"Why?" she replied as she pulled her shoes off the floor.

"I still smell dead meat."

"Shit," she muttered as she trudged off to the bathroom to sanitize her shoes.

I was back in my old form. I, of course, smelled nothing but Jenny didn't know that.

I signed back into my computer and got a message. "You have four resident charts to review and sign." What resident? I hadn't seen any patients with a resident. I asked another nurse (Jenny was still sniffing her shoes) and she told me that Dr. Hofecker was the resident that night.

"Hofucker?" I screamed. I thought I ditched him in Atlantic City.

She then volunteered that Dr. Hofecker was the son of Thomas Hofecker, the hospital administrator.

"Thomas Earhardt Hofecker II?"

"I just know him by Mr. Hofecker."

Jenny returned and proclaimed that she didn't stink. I told her I knew and giggled. I asked her about Hofucker and she motioned for me to join her in the medication room.

After we arrived safely in there and she confirmed we were alone, she said, "He is a complete ass. I think he's incompetent, but don't mess with him. His dad is a total prick. More than one physician has been fired after taking on Dr. Hofecker."

I replied to Jenny. "I know him. He is one of the dimmer bulbs in his residency program. I don't trust his judgment and I don't much trust him."

Just my freakin' luck. Not only do I have to work night shifts, which I hate, but I have to babysit Hofucker again. I can't believe he is now a third-year resident and working here. Where the hell was he all night?

Over the hours, we finally got close to caught up. I found the coffee pot and restored my caffeine levels to a functional status. Then I set out to find Hofucker. No one seemed to know where he was. People scattered when I made inquiries. I don't even know why I asked. I remembered that we had a passive tracking system in the ER that showed the location of every patient and employee.

I clicked on the screen and noted that Hofucker and a nursing assistant named Marilyn were in room 7 of POD B. The ER had three pods. All of them were open during the busiest hours. But Pods A and B were closed at night. We worked only out of Pod C.

I found the room. The door was locked. I swiped my badge at the pad, and it opened. So did my eyes. I was staring at the hairy, gyrating bare ass of Hofucker. He was standing on the stepstool at the base of a gynecological exam table. His pants were at his ankles. The feet in the stirrups had nicely painted pink nails. On the floor in front of me was a crumpled-up blue scrub suit with Marilyn's ID attached.

I closed the door and went back to my workstation in Pod C. No wonder I hadn't seen any patients with Hofucker. So why was I being asked to sign charts? I read a couple of them and realized that the patients had been discharged.

I was supposed to be seeing those patients along with the resident, not signing the chart later. In fact, when I signed the chart, I had to indicate that I examined the patient and that I was present for the most important aspects of the care of that patient. That included any procedure performed, or something to that effect. That was the only way that Medicare would pay outrageous sums for the visit. The first patient had a shoulder dislocation, received far too much sedation, and had the shoulder relocated. I confirmed with the nurse that Hofucker had done all of that without any supervision. Not good.

A few minutes later, Hofucker appeared at my side. He was far from handsome, but I had to admit that I liked looking at his face more than his ass.

"You, physician's lounge, now," he seethed.

"I don't often take orders from residents, but I think we should talk," I replied.

We retreated to the physician's lounge. Hofucker cut loose.

"We are not in AC anymore dude. I don't know who you think you are pal, but my dad is the fucking CEO here. He won't take it kindly when I tell him about your peeping Tom act."

I couldn't believe what I was hearing. This guy was practicing medicine unsupervised and then he thought it was ok to dip the wick while on duty.

"Hofucker, you are now a third-year resident. You know that you are required to be supervised. I don't sign charts of patients that I never participated in their care. Everyone here tonight busted their ass while you grabbed some. If we ever work together again, you will follow the rules. Keep your sexual escapades to yourself and out of this department. I am not averse to reporting unacceptable behavior."

"Go ahead, turn me in. My dad will squelch any crap you invent."

"I wouldn't waste my time reporting you here. I was thinking the state board of medicine and the American Board of Emergency Medicine. You do hope to get a permanent license and board certification, don't you?"

"Look you prick, you will be sorry," screamed Hofucker as he nearly broke the door down, leaving the room.

I returned to the ED where Jenny just shook her head. "Why must you rock the boat? Your first night here and all hell is breaking loose."

"Does everyone get a sex break or is that just a resident perc?" I was kind of hoping it was a Supreme Medical Center custom and that she planned to initiate me.

Unfortunately, she ignored the question. "We only have one patient left in triage. Do you want to order anything from the cafeteria?"

I asked. "Are there any good pizza places still open?"

"Giovanni's never closes. Their pizza is awesome," she said.

I smiled and replied, "Tell the staff that I am buying."

That would set me back around $50, but the goodwill it bought was invaluable. I knew that I would need all the help I could get to survive here. And I thought I had a lock on the AON money.

I got to the ward secretary and gave her enough money to order pizza for the department. I also asked her if there was any way that someone could slip across the street to Walmart. She had a break coming up and said she needed to get a birthday card. I told her what I wanted, and she laughed.

One half hour later, the ER was empty except for two drunks who were too drunk to discharge. They were on monitors and tucked away. They were no problem. When the secretary got back from Walmart, she gave me my package. I went to work. She got a nice pack of carrots. I selected a big one and then pulled up the picture of the one we extracted from the carrot dude on my phone. I carefully cut a small piece out of the fresh carrot, and it was a perfect match for one in the garbage.

We all sat down to eat in the breakroom and Jenny introduced me to the staff that I had not yet met. She was quick to include that I had insisted on buying pizza. She even mentioned that I might have half a clue about practicing emergency medicine. Suddenly, she screamed and threw the piece of pizza she had just been handed on the floor. I guessed that Jenny didn't like carrots on her pizza. Especially a carrot with a piece missing that might previously have been sexually abused.

It took ten minutes to convince her that the carrot was a fake, made to look like the other carrot. She was certain that we had put the carrot I extracted from the patient on her pizza. She was pissed but eventually she laughed and ate a different piece of pizza from a different box. I had made some new friends, which I would need more than I knew.

Carrot man walked away with the title that night and I was off to a good start. I donated the winnings to those attending the breakfast in-service at the Daily Double. At 7 AM, I gave a report to the oncoming physician about the two drunks and mentioned my concern about the supervision of the residents. I didn't mention the coital act I witnessed. He nodded but said nothing. I quickly surmised that he didn't give a shit if it didn't affect him. Tons of them in medicine. I grabbed my briefcase and headed for the door. With any luck I would be at the track before 7:30 and possibly get all my jogging and training in before noon. I can never sleep in the afternoon. Today, hopefully, would be an exception to that.

As I approached the exit door, a slightly rotund, bald, middle-aged man with a salt-and-pepper beard blocked my path. He had a pink bowtie on. I never liked anyone who wore a bowtie. My streak was going to remain intact.

"Dr. Zander?" he asked.

"Guilty as charged," I retorted.

"I need to talk to you a moment. My name is Thomas Hofecker II. I am the CEO here."

"Nice to meet you," I replied and offered my hand. I immediately nicknamed him Deuce from here on out. Hofucker the second equaled Deuce in my quick-witted head.

"Cut the bullshit!" he screamed as he motioned me into the family room.

That's the private room where we took families to give them bad news. I followed him in there and we stood eye to eye about six inches from each other's faces. He asked me to sit down, and I did. He decided to stand. No doubt some macho bullshit trick that he learned in administrator school.

"I hope you realize that you started here via the use of temporary privileges. Those are in effect until your full privileges can be processed by the credentials, executive committee, and board of directors. During this time, you have temporary privileges that can revoked by me without cause."

"Would this discussion have anything to do with me catching your son fornicating while on duty?"

"I have no idea what you are talking about," he stammered.

"The hell you don't," I said as I stood up again, face to face with him. "Look pal…" By now, you know what it means when I call someone pal. I was livid. "I don't know what your game is here. I know your son is feared in the ED and that other ED physicians who challenged him were shown the door."

"True," he smiled as he straightened that idiot bowtie.

"Well, Deuce, today your streak ends. Can I call you Deuce? Like I give a shit. You are now and forever Deuce. Your son is going to become a model citizen in the department, and you are going to see to it." I stared at him defiantly.

Deuce backed up two steps and recollected himself. "And what allows you to have this delusional thinking?" he inquired.

"You see Deuce, if you pull my privileges, you will badly screw up my life. I am trying to do something for my family that depends on me working here…"

Deuce interrupted. "That is not my problem, you are suspended. Goodbye."

He tried to walk out, but I pushed him back down in a chair.

"Now you prick, listen to me, and listen well. If I lose my privileges, I will make just one call. After that one call, you will regret what you did."

"Doctor, are you threatening me? Not only will you lose your privileges, but if I press charges, you can end up in jail. That could jeopardize your medical license. Wise up and move on."

I pulled up a chair and faced him. "Deuce, I had hoped we could work something out. But maybe I need to make that call."

Was I calling a hitman? Nah, something worse. Medicare.

"You see, I suspect that your son has been doing unsupervised work in the ED. I know this because he was mad that I would not sign his charts. Now either this is the first time that he pulled this crap, or it has been going on for a while. I don't know for sure, but I suspect it has been going on for a while. After that call to Medicare goes through, in come the inspectors and surveyors. They pull charts and talk to staff, including doctors, nurses, aids, and secretaries. If they conclude that your physicians have been signing charts claiming they supervised work done by your son that they had not supervised, your little hospital is finished. The fines and restitution will destroy you, and they will likely throw your place right out of the Medicare program. Checkmate you fat fuck. Now get out of my way, I have work to do."

Deuce looked stunned.

CHAPTER 8

Miracle Mile Racetrack and Casino

Krenshaw, NJ

0725 June 3

It was a short drive to the track. I was still fuming as I passed the security gate and headed to the barn. Mom was busy mucking out a few stalls. Stephanie was just coming up the hill from the track. She had taken Fired Up Rio for her first training mile. I should have done that, but my interlude with Deuce had put me behind.

I exited the truck, and asked Stephanie, "Well, how was she?"

You never knew what Stephanie was going to say. I was happy that no one was in earshot.

"She is a nasty bitch today. Jumpin' shadows, not paying attention, and not too interested in doin' any fucking work. I think she's horsin,' and only wants to get laid."

I got a half a smile on my face. Only Stephanie could have put a smile on my face this morning. I grabbed a blanket to put on Rio.

"Thanks for getting her started, we are going three more trips today. I hope to be out of here by noon."

There was variability in how people trained their horses. Rio was a three-year-old who hadn't raced at age two. Carl said she was immature and decided to let her grow up a little. She was making her first start of this season on Friday. Tuesday was her training day. After jogging for a few miles, she would go on one-mile trips of 3:00, 2:30, 2:15 and the last around 2:00. With about an hour off in between to cool down. Stephanie had taken her for the first trip.

I found my old helmet and got ready to find the next horse that was ready to train. I passed my mother who was maneuvering a wheelbarrow of steaming horse shit and straw up the ramp to the manure dumpster.

"Don't go!" she screamed as she dumped her load. "I have to talk to you." She parked the wheelbarrow and lit a cigarette.

"Mom, I thought you quit!" I chided her.

"The only thing I quit doing was lying about it. So, I smoke, big deal," she retorted.

Mom looked like she had aged about twenty years since Carl left. She had lost weight and was eating and sleeping poorly. It showed. She informed me that the presiding racing judge had stopped in the barn this morning. I could tell right away that this was not good news.

"What did he want?" I asked.

"He says that you can't drive this week unless you drive successfully in all three qualifying races this morning."

Mom went on to say that she had thought that my license was still good once I had turned in my updated physical. But the judges had the right to see me drive in qualifying races if they wanted, and they wanted. Although I was tired, I didn't mind getting some race condition experience in before "real" races this week. I had been training and jogging horses, but I was very nervous about being in an actual race. Doing the qualifiers this morning might help me get over some of that.

Then, Mom handed me the entry sheets for the qualifiers. I was driving three of the biggest rats the track had to offer. That's what we called racehorses that lacked talent. The first was Hubba Hubba. Five years old and still a maiden. He was 0 for 57 lifetime starts and was being forced to qualify because of repeated breaks. That was defined as a failure to maintain the required gate of the race, either trotting or pacing. He was a pacer, but he had this bad habit of breaking stride at a whim. He was known for creating confusion and even a few wrecks on the track.

If I survived that race, I then got the privilege of sitting behind Eight Ball. I had heard she was a runaway. Once the gate pulled away, she pulled away like a bat out of hell. It took all your strength to control her. Drivers were usually left with sore arms, and little or no purse money, because she could never finish the mile fast enough to win much.

The third and last piece of work was Slightly Devious. He was more than slightly. He was downright nuts and probably unsafe. I had heard that once he was in front and decided to head back to the barn, right in the middle of the race. He made a right turn in front of seven horses, and they all ended up lying on the track. Luckily no one got killed. Hopefully, I will be equally lucky.

As I continued jogging and training horses that morning, I saw a few familiar faces. But most of the people on the track were strangers. Five years is a long time in the racing business, and the faces turned over quickly. I soon realized that I hadn't forgotten how to get a horse around the track. Things were going well. Fired Up Rio completed her fourth training mile in 1:59.1 and the last quarter in 28 seconds, which was great. I had to keep her mind on her business. Stephanie was right, she was not focused today. Neither was I, so we were a good pair. Rio didn't seem tired after her last mile and ran back up the hill to the barn. I thought she was well set up for her Friday debut.

Stephanie was her usual quiet self for most of the morning but wanted to walk with me down to the paddock for the qualifiers. She tried her best to speak slowly and clearly.

"Watch your ass, there are a lot of crooked motherfuckers here who would like nothing better than to see your ass fucked."

I digested that for a moment and replied. "Look Steph, I'd like to tell you that I am my old self, and that I am ready to go. But I have to admit that I have doubts. I guess I will find out when the gate opens."

"Can I give you some advice?" she asked with those big blue eyes as intent and caring as I had ever seen.

"Sure, I am not sure it will help but go ahead."

Stephanie started chanting and bouncing up and down. You know the way Drew Brees did with the Saints before they kicked off. I grinned and thanked her for getting me ready.

"Fuck you," she answered. "Just watch and listen." She then continued to dance and scream.

"Race one

To walk away when this one is done

Keep his head up to the sun

If he looks down, he will run

Who is Moses?

Number six will lead you to the roses."

"What does that mean?" I inquired.

"Hubba likes to get his head down and every break he has made happened when he did it. It's probably some kind of choking thing. Attach your horse to the ass of the six horse and she will lead you to the winner's circle. Just like Moses led the Israelites," she blurted out as she kept dancing up and down.

"Race two

To keep your hands from turning blue

Make sure the mare knows your intentions are true

To be sure she doesn't go south

Take care of her sore mouth.

Who is Moses?

You is Moses"

After a few seconds' pause, she finished her show.

"Race three

This horse needs to see

That you got the reins

And ice water in your veins

He has to know

That you will tell him when to stop and go

Who is Moses?

The one horse is best and usually closes."

Before I could ask her another question she left and headed back to the barn. I did know two things. First, Stephanie had a gift. She knew everything about every horse on the track. She saw and remembered every quirk, every strength, and every weakness. Even though she picked an odd way to tell me, the information would be spot on. The second thing I knew is that she loved me. This was her way of getting me safely back into racing.

CHAPTER 9

Miracle Mile Racetrack and Casino

Krenshaw, NJ

1055 June 3

I only had a few minutes to get to the track. So, I ran down the hill. I quickly passed the breathalyzer station and borrowed a flak jacket from one of the judges. I got to the paddock and found my way to Hubba Hubba's stall. The trainer was waiting for me. Bill Mallory was a reasonable guy but not the friendliest or most talkative.

"Hi Bill," I said as I offered my hand.

He looked me up and down and said, "Zach you look skinny. Are you sure you are up for this?"

I answered, "I am as ready as can be. Any suggestions?"

"Don't fall off." He laughed as we walked the horse onto the track.

How rude of me to think you know all about harness racing. These are the horses with the cart (sulky) behind them. The drivers are average-sized people, not like the little people who ride thoroughbred horses. Good thing. I would have to cut off both legs and one arm if I wanted to make the weight requirements for a thoroughbred. I had a tee shirt that I loved that summed up how I had felt about racing. It showed a harness horse with the caption, "There's nothing like a thousand pounds of fun between your legs."

The horses either trot, moving diagonal legs at the same time, like your cat. Or they pace, where they move legs on the same side of their body at the same time. In that case they kind of waddle. The good ones waddle really fast. Almost all the races are at a distance of one mile. Since our track here is ⅝ mile, they go around a little less than one and a half times. The starting gate is mounted to the back of the car or truck and leads the horses to the starting line. By the time we reach the start, the car is moving around thirty-five miles per hour. At the start line, the car pulls away and the race begins.

This is where the first major decision must be made. Do I go for the lead or try to come from behind? It's usually better to be near the front of the pack. But if you make your horse work too hard, too early, they might not have much energy left at the end of the race. Once you make that decision, you have to get to the pylons as soon as possible.

There used to be a rail at the inside of the racecourse. But that left horses that broke stride no place to bail out. A few years ago, most US tracks removed the rail and put in place pylons that the horses had to stay inside of. But they could duck inside the pylons if they broke stride to avoid a wreck. It was much safer and avoided many accidents.

Back to the racing action, you can stay to the outside if you want. But you lose around fifty feet for each of the three turns if you are not at the pylons. It is very difficult to win doing that. Once you settle in then you must decide when you want to make your move. Come out too early, and your horse could tire. Wait too long and the front runners can get pretty far ahead, making it difficult to catch up. Or you can get boxed in.

A lot of this is like NASCAR. There is a certain amount of drafting. Sitting in the two-hole position (at the rail behind the leader) is usually pretty good. You get covered up from the wind, but you are close enough to make a late move. That is provided the horse on the lead is a Moses and carries you to the top of the stretch. If the lead horse is rat, and stops in front of you, it could ruin any chance you have of winning. You always need to know who you are following.

At some point, you have to decide if you want to be the first one to pull out of line and head toward the front. This position is called first-up or first-over. Ideally you don't want to be in this position for more than one turn because you must go a longer distance. You are not against the pylons anymore. Depending on the horse and the race, it is sometimes better to follow the first-over horse. This is called the second-over position. You get the benefit of drafting behind the first-over horse, but you still are going a little extra distance.

I mentioned NASCAR before. Driving a racehorse is like taking a race car around the track with one gallon of gas. You got to be careful how you use it. Leave out of the gate too fast, and you could be out of gas by the half-mile pole. Starting and stopping your horse burns up energy (their gas) and leads to lost races. A nice, smooth, well-paced effort will get you the farthest.

As we neared the track, I grabbed Hubba Hubba's lines and jumped in the race bike. We walked onto the track for a short warm-up score and then we had to get behind the gate. We drew the three-hole, and it was my job to have him in the correct position. He seemed pretty interested and looked to be pacing soundly. I got him up behind the gate, and it started. I was sweating like a whore in church. My heart was beating about two hundred times a minute, and I was hyperventilating. This was no good, I needed to pull up.

Actually, I needed a paper bag to breathe into, but I had none. Plus, I didn't have a free hand to hold it. In my mind, the video of the accident was playing over and over, with my face getting stepped on every time. That's when I saw them. Stephanie and Mom were standing at the railing of the paddock with a big sign that said, "Good luck ZZ." I slowed my breathing down and suddenly Stephanie's poem crept into my head.

Race one

To walk away when this one is done

Keep his head up to the sun

If he looks down, he will run

Who is Moses?

Number six will lead you to the roses.

By now, we were about 50 yards to the starting line. Hubba Hubba had his head down and I gently pulled up on the lines. The next thing I knew, we were on the gate and nearing the start line. As the gate pulled away, I spoke to the horse and let him leave the gate. He got to the pylons and was in the lead until the six-horse pulled out and passed us. No big deal, we were following Moses. Hubba Hubba was relaxed and so was I. We got a nice ride around the track. Around the last turn the three-horse pulled up beside us and was pacing well but not fast enough to pass the six.

Hubba Hubba was still live. I lifted his head a little higher in the air and switched leads as we entered the stretch. I wanted to pull to the outside but the three-horse was still out there. About fifty feet into the stretch, a lane opened on the inside of the lead horse that only trailing horses were allowed to use. We bid our time and I pulled left as we hit the lighting lane. Hubba Hubba was a little tentative. I don't think he had ever been this close to the lead and didn't know what to do. I ran my whip over the crown of his ass, and he grabbed the bit a little harder. He started to gain on the six-horse. The driver of the six went to the whip as I used a couple wrist flips to ask Hubba to dig in. He responded well and we hit the finish line at the same time as the six. It was a photo, and we lost by a nose.

I slowed the horse down and we turned around to head back to the paddock. Bill Mallory was running on the sidewalk outside the track and screaming.

"Holy shit, holy shit, you almost won. He looked like a racehorse!! Will you drive him for me next week?"

I screamed back, "Sure if I don't have one of our horses in!"

"Thanks ZZ, I owe you," Bill replied.

I walked into the paddock to find only a groom with Eight Ball. The horse looked alright, but the groom looked like he was high on heroin or something. Small, squinty eyes and a stupid look on his face. No wonder this horse had trouble. She probably never got fed right or cared for properly. I was going to need help here and hopefully Stephanie's poem would have some answers.

Race two

To keep your hands from turning blue

The second we hit the track the mare sped off. My first intention was pull back hard on the reins. But if she had a sore mouth like Stephanie had surmised then she would fight that. The war would be on. I let her move around the turn and ever so gently, I pulled back a little on the reins. Then I pointed her in the direction of the barn. She had to slow down to make that turn, but she wanted to go home. As she slowed to nearly a walk, I spun her away from the track exit. She was jogging lightly now, and I eased up on the lines. The more I relaxed, the more she relaxed. We got back behind the starting gate, and I turned and put her nose on the gate. She was pushing at the gate because she wanted to go faster. I let the lines loosen, and she figured out that she couldn't push the gate down. She relaxed.

As the gate pulled away, I held the lines firmly as I chirped to her. She left the gate with purpose and quickly gained the lead. I knew that no one would pull on us because she had always been on the front. It was suicide for anyone who tried too early to take the lead. I also knew that no driver had been able to rate her. That was to get her to slow her speed down to last longer. Many of my girlfriends had tried to rate me. I digress. Like me, Eight Ball usually went flat out until she quit. Most often, that was around the ¾ pole. Well today I tightened up on the lines while trying to be as gentle as possible. She must have sensed that I was on her side. She slowed a little and relaxed more.

We got to the quarter a little faster than I wanted but halftime was perfect. The five-horse came first over down the backside. Everyone figured Eight Ball was getting ready to quit. At the ¾ pole, I let her completely loose and sat back. She had a great kick and opened a three-length lead that she never gave up. Eight Ball had won the qualifier and found out that racing could be fun. The groom looked shocked but was still so stoned that he didn't quite grasp the importance of this. I was grinning from ear to ear. I saw Mom at the rail on the way back to the paddock, and I told her to try to buy Eight Ball. As it turned out, the owners were more than happy to unload her. She bought her for five thousand dollars. I was going to have to pull a lot of carrots out of dark places to pay for her. But with a little help and a lot of love, I knew she could make money. I also knew we could give her a better home.

Time for the last poem:

Race three

This horse needs to see

That you got the reins

And ice water in your veins

He must know

That you will tell him when to stop and go

Who is Moses

The one horse is best and usually closes.

On to Slightly Devious. This horse looked squirrely. Beady eyes and a dumb look. He was big and muscular.

All the trainer told me was, "be careful, he can be unpredictable."

Thanks, pal. What the hell, the life insurance is paid up, and if worse comes to worse, Mom can use the money, I mused. As I tried to get on the bike, the horse suddenly sped up and almost dumped me out of the bike. I barely got into the seat, and then he reared up. He was standing on his back legs. The only thing you can do when that happens is throw the lines at the horse. If you pull back on them, they can fall right back onto your lap. At a thousand pounds per horse, I could do without that.

I threw the lines at the horse and slid off the sulky. He came back to the ground. I walked up to his face and got about one inch from one of his beady eyes. I just stared. He blinked, and then I jumped back on the bike. He pulled like he wanted to take off, but I pulled back so hard

I thought I was going to break his neck. He stopped, and I slowly let the lines out. He then paced on normally, and we got in line for the race. It was a battle of wills, and I won the first round.

We had the five-hole. I shook the lines as the gate left, and he sped to the lead. He let me control him, and we got a reasonable quarter. He was moving nicely as we neared the half-mile pole. He then suddenly jerked to the right, in the direction of the ramp to the barn. And in a millisecond, I knew what was going on. By then, he had gone down on both front knees and was ready to cause a wreck of the entire field. I pulled up on the lines as hard as I could. I almost stood in the stirrups of the race bike. He bounced up from the track and resumed pacing. Two horses directly behind him broke stride, but no one went down. We got passed by the one horse who won the race and finished third. But we finished, and neither one of us was lying on the track.

One of the assistant judges came down to the paddock and told the trainer that Slight Devious was barred from the track. He would have to go elsewhere to race. He was too dangerous to be allowed to race here. I asked the judge if I was qualified to race. He said that since Slightly Devious was not qualified, neither was I. I could have one more chance in a month if I wanted, but he wanted to see more of me. I had heard that this judge was dirty and that he was in bed with one of the bigger barns. He was asshole buddies with the top driver at the track. Billie "cha-ching" Browner.

I called the presiding judge, Mike Dalton, who came down to the track.

"Will," he said to the other judge, "why is Zach not qualified?"

Will looked at the ground as he answered. "You saw the last race. It was only sheer luck that all the horses and drivers weren't hurt. We can't have that kind of driving here."

Mike frowned and said, "Now, Will, you know as well as I do that this horse is a nut. We should have tossed him months ago. Today Zach saved us the embarrassment of that mistake coming to light. Only a highly skilled driver could have kept that horse from falling in front of the field. Zach, as presiding judge, I am overriding Will and qualifying you. See you this week."

Stephanie and Mom had the barn chores done and all of the horses put away. I was dreaming of getting some sleep as we drove home. We relived the three races, and I complimented Stephanie on her knowledge of the horses.

"How did you know so much about the horses I drove?" I asked as we drove home.

"I know every horse on that track. The ones that ship in I have to watch a bit, but even they aren't too difficult to figure out. They talk to me, and I talk to them."

I pondered that as we arrived back home. One last job before hitting the sack. Sick call at the school. Our cost-cutting had forced us to cut out the services of a great nurse practitioner who managed sick calls for us. I got volunteered. No big deal but I was getting pretty tired. Luckily today, we had only two patients. One with an earache and another who was repeatedly soiling his pants. The diagnoses were simple, but the exams were not.

Most kids don't like to be examined, and some special needs kids are especially difficult. After about ten minutes of talking, and Stephanie intervening, the exam of the earache was done. Two clicks of the computer and the antibiotic needed was ordered and would be delivered by the pharmacy.

The pooper was a little more difficult because I wanted to do a rectal exam—our patient did not. That negotiation took forty minutes, but it paid off. I found a large fecal impaction that needed broken apart. The poor little guy had encopresis. Not to be confused with an enchilada, encopresis was a child repeatedly soiling himself. One of the causes was a fecal impaction that stopped the passage of stool. The result was diarrhea that went around the blockage and into the drawers of the unlucky child. After the rectal exam, I thought that the little guy hated me. But when he kept the same clothes on for more than two hours, he might change his mind. I know his caretakers will be happy.

CHAPTER 10

Fired Up Farms
Krenshaw, NJ
1655 June 4

My second shift had gone ok. I arrived a little early, and that pleased Jenny to no end. No one died that shouldn't have. Dawn, one of the RNs, grabbed the AON money with a gutsy bet on a drug seeker who faked a kidney stone. She caught him pricking his finger and adding a few drops of blood to his urine sample. I thought someone would beat that, but it was one of those nights where most patients and families were legitimate. Pretty unusual occurrence.

Also unusual was how well things ran at the barn this morning. Mom, Stephanie, and I got everything done in an amazing time. The vet, feed supply vendor, and our blacksmith were all on time and that was very unusual. At 11:30 AM, I finished stacking the bags of feed and headed home. Mom and Stephanie had a few more chores to get done but even they would get home early.

I was planning on studying the racetrack program when I got home. But the bed was so comfortable, and I was so tired that I succumbed to a deep slumber. I woke up when Stephanie pounded on the door and screeched. "Get the fuck up, get the fuck up." It was five o'clock, and I had to be at the track by six to blow the breathalyzer. Maybe I could blow the guy running the breathalyzer and get more sleep. No such luck. Unfortunately, I was in the first, second, and tenth races. I trudged into the shower and tried to wake up my tired mind and body.

I had the program in my hand as I arrived in the kitchen with just enough time to gulp down some dinner. Too bad I couldn't take my time. Mom was an exceptional cook, and Swiss steak was one of her best dishes. Stephanie looked indignant as I opened the program.

"Fuck you. Don't you trust me?" she asked with those sad blue eyes that no one could resist.

"Of course, I do. But I still need to be ready for these races," I answered.

"Then eat and be ready, I got this," Stephanie added with a grin.

Tonight, I was driving three of our horses. In the first race was Fired Up Blossom. She was a trotting filly with some talent. She was in a race for filly trotters that had won two but not more than three races. She was supposedly easy to drive but didn't seem to have much guts. Great, another pet to drive around the track.

The second race brought Boom Boom Boom. I know, you thought all our horses were named Fired Up something. Well, the ones that we bred were. The ones that we bought as yearlings were, but the others were not. Once a horse raced with a name, you weren't allowed to change it. So, anything we bought or claimed after it had raced for a purse, we were stuck with their name. My mom had claimed Boom Boom Boom last week for $15,000.

A claiming race is a race in which every horse in there is for sale. If you owned a horse at the track, you could buy them for the claiming price. My mom had spent $15,000 for her. Tonight, she was in races for $20,000 horses. If she got claimed, we would make $5,000, but the competition would be tougher. It was going to be an uphill battle to win.

In the tenth race, I had Fired Up Leah. She was three and still a maiden, meaning she never won a race. She had only raced five times as a two-year-old and three times this year at three. She was a nervous horse and Stephanie had been working with her at the farm. To this point, she did not look too promising.

Mom left early for the track, and Stephanie and I went in my truck. I was dead tired but anxious about the races. Stephanie was Stephanie—excited, on the bit, and raring to go.

"I love you ZZ," she said.

"I love you too Stephanie, you know that."

"I do. So, you have to believe in me."

"Of course, I do." I nodded.

"Then listen up. Here's the scoop.

Blossom lacks guts

But she has speed

Show her how to use it for what she needs

Who is Moses?

The three

Boom Boom Boom was a good buy

Don't let anyone look her in the eye

Who is Moses?

You is."

She took a breath and went on.

"Leah is a beast

First or second at the least

Get her to settle down

Then ride her hard and not like a clown

She knows what she got

Let her roll and roll a lot."

We got to the track, and things got crazy. I had to sign a bunch of papers and get to the breathalyzer box. Of course, I passed. Who in the hell had time for a drink? I didn't. Then, I had to jog the horses for the first two races. As I came back into the paddock with Boom Boom Boom, I found Stephanie with her fists up. She had squared off against a groom for the leading stable. I handed off Boom Boom Boom to her groom and grabbed Stephanie around the waist.

Then I found out what this was all about. Johnny Joe Fuzznuts from the Supreme Stable (not his name, but that's what Stephanie called him) said that I was a pussy because I quit racing after a little accident. Stephanie took exception to that and was prepared to kick his ass. Because we had races to run and money to make, I couldn't let her do that. But I had to love her. This was going to be a battle, but I had to like my team.

After the national anthem and lots of calming words to Stephanie, there was the call to the post for the first race. I walked beside Blossom as we headed to the track. I was surprisingly calm. I did not give a shit anymore about getting hurt, but I was very nervous about the money.

Blossum was calm in the post-parade, which made sense for a horse lacking courage. But Stephanie had told me that she had speed and that I should use that for what she needed. The lights went on, and I knew immediately what I needed to do.

We had the five-hole and eased out of the gate. I managed to secure a position at the pylons in the sixth spot. We reached the half in a leisurely fifty-eight seconds, and I decided to let her go. I popped the earplugs, eased up on the reins, and she took off.

"Now 5th, now 4th, now 3rd, now 2nd," bellowed the announcer as we worked our way first over up the backside.

Soon, we were side by side with the leading horse, Pepper Grinder. He was driven by none other than Billie "Cha-ching" Browner, the top driver at the track. I called him ba ba ba ba Billie? He had a terrible speech impediment. Normally, I am sympathetic to that stuff, but I knew that he was very sensitive, and I wanted to get him fired up.

Billie and I had been close, once. Carl and Mom were good to him. He started as a groom for us. Eventually under Carl's tutelage, he got his license. It took about a year for him to show his potential. Once he climbed the driver's ladder, he forgot who my parents were. With great urging, he would drive an occasional horse for us. But he started to hang out with the "wrong crowd" at the track. When I was injured, he signed an exclusive arrangement with Supreme Stables. They used him as much as possible, and he could drive for no one else. Supreme Stables, Supreme Medical, was that a coincidence? There are no coincidences.

All that aside I found myself side by side with an old friend. Being the affable soul that I am, I looked over at him and smiled as I greeted him. "Ba ba ba ba Billie!"

"Fa Fa Fa Fa Fuck you," he shouted back. He drifted his horse out toward me, and we briefly rubbed wheels.

"Are you really as dumb as you look?" I shouted as I steadied my horse.

Blossum was a little intimidated by a horse being that close to her, and she started to slow down. Pepper Grinder opened a half-length lead.

"EEEEEEAAAAT SHHHITTT," chuckled Billy.

I pulled Blossum's earplugs and reefed her one on her big brown ass. Around the turn, she passed Pepper Grinder. We pulled back in front of Billie as we entered the home stretch. I drove Blossum down the lane, and she started to pull away. I was praying that I hadn't lost my touch. I worked up a nice wad of spit in my mouth, leaned my head back, and let that saliva fly. My aim was true, and my distance was perfectly calculated. The hocker of the century just missed his horse's head and hit Billie in the face as we crossed the wire.

The parts of his face that weren't covered in my saliva and snot were red. He was stuttering all kinds of shit at me as we pulled our horses up around the turn. I headed back to the winner's circle, and he went to the paddock to get the next horse he was racing. Stephanie and Mom met me in the winner's circle for a picture.

Mom said, "Great drive, your horse paid $30 to win (for a $2 bet). Too bad you didn't bet her."

"I didn't bet her, but Pisscatcher did." I smiled.

I had him put $100 to win on Blossum that was now worth $1500. We still had a long way to go to get to $6 million, but we were off and racing.

Boom Boom Boom jumped out to an easy lead in her race but tired badly around the last turn and finished last.

"Mom, better get her scoped. She must have bled and might need Lasix," I said as I quickly handed the reins to her.

I had bet $200 on her and now I was only $1200 ahead, minus whatever I decided to tip PC. As I walked back to the paddock for the next race, I spied Billie leaning against the door to the drivers' lounge. Although I preferred not to interact with him, I had no choice but to walk past him to get to my horse.

In his best attempt at a coherent sentence, he smiled and said, "Do do do you fuck u u u your hor hor hor whore sister? Ev ev ev ev every one else does".

I reached back with my left arm to get a good swing at the little bastard. Suddenly, something grabbed my arm and nearly broke it off. The hand that grabbed me was the size of a basketball, and the skin was thick and tough.

I looked around to see Amos Weaver, the farrier, ready to pull off my arm like a turkey drumstick. Amos was a farrier, not a fairy. He was a blacksmith. He was 6 foot 2 inches. That was 74 inches tall of pure muscle. His arms were like dumbbells. His muscles stole most of the blood badly needed by his pea sized brain. He was owned and operated by the Supreme Stables. Luckily the presiding judge came around the bend, and Amos let go of my arm.

In passing, the presiding judge advised me that the next time I felt the need to clear my throat during a race, it would cost me $500.

"Yes sir," I replied. I could have sworn that I saw half a smile on his face.

I worked my way to Fired Up Leah as they bugled us for the post-parade. No one said a word as we walked to the track. Leah was a little feisty but settled down as we walked onto the track. We had the eight-hole and were following our old friend Billie, who was driving GaGa Gangster from the seven-hole. As the announcer introduced the horses, I heard that Billie's horse was owned by Supreme Stables. Then I saw him. Standing at the rail with binoculars around his neck was an asshole wearing a bowtie. It was Deuce, aka Thomas Earhardt Hofecker II. As it turns out, he was one of the two principal owners of Supreme Stables. I tried to wave at my new friend, but somehow, only my middle finger went up; Amos must have hurt me more than I knew.

I was hoping that Leah would get out of the gate well and secure a position near the front. As the gate pulled away, she just kind of floated out of the gate. We got away eighth, dead last.

As we rounded the first turn, I heard the announcer say, "And Fired Up Leah can see them all."

I considered just letting her take the night off and race her harder next week. But Stephanie had told me she was a beast, and that I should let her roll and roll a lot. I pulled to the outside and we rocketed up first over to be fourth. Just then, Sam Reston pulled his horse in front of us. I jerked Leah up in the air, and to the outside to avoid hitting him. Leah broke stride, and I had to pull back on her to get her on gait.

By the time I got her straightened out, the field had passed us by. We finished last. I filed an objection against Sam, but the judge's camera angle didn't show the infraction to be as serious as it was. They allowed him to remain second to Billie, who had won the race. I would later come to learn that Sam was the bastard son of Amos. He was also controlled and operated by Supreme Shitheads. I suspected those scumbags were cheating on almost every race. Little did I know how right I was. I knew Sam had pulled out and fouled me on purpose to let Billie's horse win.

I blew $500 betting on Leah. By the time I gave Pisscatcher $100, I only had $600 profit for the night. I was starting to think I was Always Hope's evil twin, No Hope. Maybe the ER will be quiet tonight. I am pretty tired. One win and two last-place finishes did little to wake me up.

CHAPTER 11

Emergency Department
Supreme Medical Center
Krenshaw, NJ
2355 June 4

The ER was anything but quiet. The waiting room wasn't too bad, but most of the treatment rooms were filled. I changed into my scrubs, grabbed a coffee, and prepared to dig in. Just then, I heard a scream and a crash in our radiology suite. I ran back to see a woman beating the shit out of a guy on the floor. A petite x-ray tech tried to pull the aggressor off, but she got swatted away like a fly. I stepped into the fracas and just barely ducked a punch destined for my big nose. This was a really pissed-off lady. Luckily, my experience with horses trying to strike at me in the stall paid off. I got her by the throat and pulled her off the poor guy. I was shocked to hear him motherf... me for hurting his wife. His wife?

Luckily, the police arrived and separated them before they could separate me. They had been in a huge domestic fight and were both taken to the ER. By policy, they were placed in opposite sections of the ER. Unfortunately, they both required X-rays. You guessed it, they got called to x-ray at the same time and reunited there. Never a dull moment.

Before I could sign into the computer, I heard a call for a Code Purple in room eleven. That was our signal for a psychiatric emergency, and it meant that someone was in danger. I ran back to room eleven and saw a very large man screaming into Jenny's face. He was ranting about the planets lining up and that Barack Obama was a Martian. I always wondered about that birth certificate of his. Jenny looked scared. I was terrified. An elderly security guard arrived along with one of our male aids with a cast on his arm. Taking this dude down was very likely to get some, or all of us, hurt. Unfortunately, the bookies made our staff long odds versus this mountain of a patient.

I have no idea why I did it, but I walked right up to the big dude and looked him straight in the Adam's apple. I wanted to stare into his eyes, but he was a full foot taller than me.

I said very calmly, "Sir, what is your name?"

He said, "Excelsior."

So, I took my shot, "Ok Excelsior, you are out of control. I want you to lay down on that stretcher right now so we can get you under control."

I couldn't believe it when he walked over to the stretcher and lay down. The team calmly put restraints on all four extremities. I ordered a large injection of Ativan and Haldol. A psychiatrist buddy of mine once told me that that combination could stop an elephant. I ordered up an elephant dose and Jenny jabbed him. Fifteen minutes later, he was asleep. I think he slept for the next thirty-six hours. Lucky bastard, I needed about four hours of sleep, and he got nine times that. Jenny was more than grateful, and I earned the reputation as a serious ER doc.

I finally signed in and finished "Excelsior's" chart. A few minutes later, I completed the paperwork that would plant him in the psychiatric unit for a few days. I breezed through a couple kids with fever, followed by a dude with a drip coming from his crank. Gonorrhea. Mr. G. shuddered at the thought. I looked up as I heard some noise coming from the medication room. There, I saw three nurses clapping and dancing. That was their tradition when they prepared meds for someone with gonorrhea, also known affectionally as the clap. Sickies! But I did have to laugh.

An hour later I just about had the place cleared out. A patient had arrived a few minutes ago and was screaming in agony. I saw them pushing him down the hall, and he looked to have a dislocated shoulder. I asked one of the nurses to start an IV and to give the poor dude some Dilaudid to kill the pain, and then get an x-ray. I loved to reduce shoulder dislocations.

Jenny came over to my desk and asked me to hit the pause button on the Dilaudid.

"Why?" I asked.

Jenny went on to explain. "This dude is bad news. I have seen him on at least four occasions with the same shoulder dislocation. I think he's a drug seeker. Other ER docs had to give him massive doses of narcotics to get his shoulder relocated."

I asked the nurse to hold the Dilaudid as I reviewed his records. The last time, he was treated by Hofucker, who gave him a total of 10 mg of Ativan and 500 mcg of fentanyl—massive doses. Dumbass Hofucker documented that every time he gave him a dose of medicine and tried to relocate the arm, the guy would scream and demand more medications. Of course, Hofucker just kept obliging him. That was one of the charts that he asked me to sign. Thank God I didn't because it was chock full of medical mistakes. But I noted that it was signed by another ER doc. He wasn't even on duty that night! This place was beyond crooked.

Now, drug seekers and emergency rooms go hand in hand. They usually came in with back pain, fake kidney stones, migraine headaches, or toothaches. Not that everyone who had these problems was a drug seeker. Most patients were legit, but these are some of the complaints that drug seekers commonly use. They picked something that would hurt but had few findings on the exam. I had seen thousands, but I never had one masquerading as a shoulder dislocation. But the others were mostly looking for pills, and this guy wanted potent intravenous stuff. Just my luck, a drug seeker on steroids! Unfortunately for him, I knew that anyone who dislocated their arm frequently could usually put it back in themselves, or with a little help. The ligaments are shot, so often, the shoulder goes back in easily.

I went to examine this guy, and I knew right away that he was tonight's winning patient. I thought about stepping out to make my AON wager, but Amos had already claimed him in triage. You got to get up early to get ahead of Amos. As I was mentally lamenting how much money Amos was about to pocket, the patient screamed and demanded

IV pain medication. I tried to examine his arm, and he took a swing at me with the other arm. Then the threats started.

"I will sue you and this hospital." Blah blah blah.

I really hated it when people threatened to sue. Any asshole can sue, but can you win? The nurse arrived with the IV. I whispered to her to get me 1mg of Ativan and 200mg of SUX. She smiled and left. The patient continued to rant until she came back into the room. He asked what she had in the syringes. She told him that she had Ativan in the first. He proclaimed that he usually needs 10 mg.

This being an intelligent nurse, she said, "That's great because that's exactly what I have."

I don't normally condone lying to patients, but this was one of those exceptions. She injected the medications. He closed his eyes and prepared to get nice and high. When he didn't get high immediately, he tried to say something and couldn't speak. He couldn't move a muscle.

That's when I said, "Better living through biochemistry."

I grabbed his arm and easily put it back into place. Then I used a bag-valve-mask to breathe gently for him for the next eight minutes. The nurse checked his vital signs and documented that his oxygen remained at 100%. Jenny placed his arm in a sling. Soon thereafter, he started to breathe and swear. He bitched about how painful his arm was and how he needed more medicine. Of course, more suing threats filled the air.

Some people just can't take a joke. He did get 1mg of Ativan, but instead of a massive dose of narcotic, he got a paralyzing dose of succinylcholine. Once he was paralyzed, I put the shoulder in and assisted his breathing until the medication wore off. No free high tonight, dipshit. He was still carrying on when I got right beside his ear and whispered. He shut right up and never said another word. He had a ride home and was discharged in a wheelchair.

I walked back to the nurse's station to see the entire night shift standing and applauding.

"What?" I said.

One of the nurses wanted to know what I said.

"Pretty simple. I told him that we were on to him. He got a sedative and a paralyzing drug but no narcotics. Never again would he get a narcotic from me in this ER. I also told him that if he left and never returned that I would not call other local ER's and report his game. Not wanting to be without narcs, he decided to cut his losses. We won't see him again until all the other ER's shut him off. That should be a while."

The unit secretary asked if calling the other ERs was a HIPPA Violation. (You know that law about sharing medical information that Clinton passed so no one would find out about his bent dick.)

"Of course," I said. "That's why I didn't call. Plus, I wanted the asshole to have someplace else to go instead of here. Let them figure him out!!"

Another round of applause. Amos got paid off early tonight. There could be no others to match this guy, and everyone knew it.

The last patient to be seen was an elderly lady from a nursing home with a possible elbow fracture. She fell off the toilet. Her elbow was massively swollen and deformed. She did not seem to be able to speak. She bleated like a sheep but did appear to be in great pain. A quick x-ray confirmed a fracture dislocation of the elbow.

"Who's on call for orthopedic surgery?" I asked as I walked to the nurse's station.

"I Need," replied Wanda, the secretary. Wanda and I bonded after she bought the carrot for Jenny.

"Oh Dr. Morehead." I had nick-named him "I Need," as in "I need more head." Of course, the night shift staff readily adopted my nickname for him.

Bad luck. It was about 4 AM, and I Need was notorious for not wanting to come in at night. I really thought this lady needed to have the fracture dislocation reduced. I hadn't done any elbows in a while. As expected, when I called I Need, he appeared to be near comatose.

I Need mumbled, "Admit her, sedate her, and I will see her after I do my morning cases."

I hung up, not quite sure what to do. I Need probably would not see her until at least noon. This sheep may not make it that far. I was worried about her circulation and a possible compartment syndrome.

"Jenny, get some ortho weights and some Kling wrap."

"Really??" she pouted. "I am beat. Get the lady a good whack of morphine and let I Need take care of her tomorrow. Quit trying to save the world. You do know Dr. Morehead is on the board of directors?"

"So what? No guts, no glory. Weights please."

Two nurses came back with me to the room. Granny got some nice sedation, and we placed her on her stomach. I applied the Kling wrap around her wrist and attached the metal holder. Once I was sure that the added weight would not cut off her circulation, I began to add weights, one pound at a time. A little more sedation and granny was cutting some major zzzz's. I added one more weight, and bammo, I heard a crunch of bone. We turned her over and sat her up. Her arm looked more like an arm. A confirmatory x-ray showed that her dislocation had been reduced, and her fracture was aligned well. A double win.

I pounded my chest like Tarzan. Amos laughed his ass off, and Jenny just shook her head in disbelief. I finished writing Granny's admitting orders and fell fast asleep at the desk. I think I had been out for a couple hours when Jenny woke me.

"I Need is in the nurse's station, and he wants to see you."

I finger-combed my hair and slowly walked over to the monitor he was staring at.

"Did you reduce this?" Dr. Morehead asked, pointing to Granny's X-ray.

"Yes sir, I used some mild sedation and weights, it was pretty easy."

"Well, that is damn fine work son. Most of your fellow ER docs wouldn't touch something like this. And as you say, it's not that difficult. Thanks for doing that. Her x-ray was much worse than I thought. I should have come right in."

Wow, ortho never admits to having to come in.

"Glad to help." I didn't know what else to say.

"I owe you one Dr. Zander." He reached out his hand, and I shook it.

"Call me ZZ."

"OK ZZ, in the future, if you really need me to come in, just say it. 'I Need, you have to come in.'"

"But, but, but…" I stammered. Crap. My damn nicknames were about to get me booted out of here. First, I pissed off Deuce, the CEO, and now a board member.

He just laughed. "I know you nicknamed me I Need. Funniest thing I've ever heard out of this department."

CHAPTER 12

Daily Double Bar

Krenshaw, NJ

0710 June 10

I won the AON money again last night. There was a three-night carryover, so the purse was generous. The smell of gasoline and the sound of a coughing child interrupted my trek to the coffee pot at 2 AM. I took a chance and threw my money down before anyone got the story.

I won on the brain-dead mother, not the kid. Kids were off limits from AON wagering. We did have some standards, albeit low. As it turns out, the mother found head lice on her child and decided that a home remedy of a gasoline shampoo was in order. The poor kid got sick from the fumes and coughed her brains out. After missing a few hours of sleep due to the coughing, her mom decided to bring her in. Thank God Mom wasn't a smoker, or the kid could have been barbecued.

An hour and three shampoos later, the gasoline odor was gone. Mom was given a prescription for a head lice shampoo and a stern lecture about the evils of using petroleum products for medicinal purposes. Before the vote at 6:30 AM I had to survive a claim of foul by Amos, of all people. He objected to my being in the triage area. It was a close vote, but he was overruled. I pocketed the cash.

Stephanie had texted me that she had things at the track under control and that I could go straight home. I decided to build some rapport with the ER staff. I joined them for an eye-opener at the Daily Double. Eight of us bellied up to the bar. Two drinks and a half hour later, Jenny and I were the only two left.

"Would you be able to give me a ride home?" Jenny asked. "My car is in the shop and my apartment is on your way home."

"Sure, do you want to go somewhere for breakfast?"

Jenny said, "How about I make you some breakfast? I make a terrific omelet."

"Sounds good to me," I said.

Jenny's apartment was in a nice location. The building appeared relatively new and well-managed. She was on the top floor. We (she) decided it was a good idea to walk up the steps for exercise. I could have done without it, but I was hungry and thirsty.

Her apartment was tastefully decorated. She led me to the balcony. I was about to secure a seat in an extremely comfortable-looking lounge chair. It was a clear morning, and it was nice to be smelling fresh-cut grass and looking at well-manicured landscaping instead of a horse's ass.

Before I could sit down, Jenny said, "Would you mind taking a shower. I can still smell the gasoline on you. I have some fresh scrubs."

That Jenny didn't mince words. She handed me a towel and fresh scrubs and pointed me to the bathroom. I sniffed my pits. I didn't smell any gasoline. What did she get a whiff of?

"Can I get you a beer, or would you prefer a Bloody Mary?" she asked as she kicked off her shoes.

"I'll take a beer, IPA if you have one."

Five minutes later I got out of the shower to find a beautifully poured beer in a frosted mug sitting on the bathroom vanity. It was adorned with a generous slice of fresh orange. I chugged half of it and headed for the balcony.

Life was good, and then it got better. That damn Jenny had taken the seat I was craving in the chaise lounge chair. But in the process of sitting down all her clothes fell off. There must have been a wind gust. That woke up Mr. Gadoonga, who had his breakfast before I did. Rat bastard, I was hungry. But he hadn't been fed in a while, so I let it pass.

The omelet was excellent too, when I got around to eating. Jenny wanted to go into the second inning and what could I do? She fed me. But at the bottom of the second, I had to head for home.

On the way home, I pondered what had just happened. Mr. G was very tired and incredibly happy. I was tired and happy too, but I worried about the ramifications of diddling the nurse manager of my ER. Those workplace relationships could be a pain in the ass. Mr. G assured me it would be ok if it happened frequently. He is such a comfort, and a total pig. Plus, it was seventy-five miles each way to see Bella. Think of the savings on gas.

CHAPTER 13

Emergency Department
Supreme Medical Center
Krenshaw, NJ
2345 June 30

Life was good. I was dipping the wick on a regular basis. I had risen to be the number two driver at the track. I was picking up live drives from different trainers each night. We were still short of money, but I was starting to build a war chest.

Stephanie and I had shortened our analysis of each race, so she didn't have to dance up and down and make rhymes. Sometimes it was just one word, like "chooch." That meant I needed to take the lead and not give it up. Or she would say "position, first five." That meant leave the gate for position and pull first over to follow the five horse. Last was "duck and good luck." That meant I was to pull the horse off the gate and try to make my best move. With her guidance I won a lot of races that I might not have on my own.

Fired Up Rio won her first race by a neck. She raced well but was a little lazy coming down the stretch. It was as if she was waiting on the other horses to catch her. I asked Stephanie to try some different head and eye equipment to allow her to see more or less.

She also told me something that might have been helpful to know before the race. Rio had a quirk. All horses have them. A good trainer can figure them out. But Rio was kind of a masochist. Most times, she went about her business. But if she started to swish her tail and slow down, you had to hit her with the whip. It was as if Rio was demanding it, Stephanie explained. When Rio did it during training miles, Stephanie would whack her until she quit swishing, or the mile was over.

"What if you don't use the whip?" I asked. I hated to use a whip, and I often did not race with one.

"She will stick 'em in." That was Stephanie speak for Rio will make a break. "Trust me, she does this all the time. She only got to the races when I figured it out."

Work in the ER was pretty good too. For some reason Jenny was in a lot better mood lately. I came to know a lot of the staff and I really enjoyed working with those sick bastards. I had become particularly fond of Amos. He was a paramedic that worked part time in the ER in addition to running with his crew. He was very observant and intuitive. He could smell bullshit coming a mile away and he usually deflected it. I liked his style, plus he was a hell of a worker. Night shift staffing was not generous. One or two slackers could kill you. I was always glad to see Amos' name on the schedule.

The drug seeker with the bum shoulder hadn't been back in a few weeks. The staff thought I was a genius. Jenny even asked me to present an in-service to the nurses. She had thought that I could review triage procedures with them. I was happy to do it, although she may not have been as thrilled when it was over.

I arrived early tonight for the in-service and Jenny met me at the door. Fortunately, the ER was not that busy. We were able to get most staff into the conference room for the presentation. Jenny had even arranged to video the session for other shifts to view at their leisure. She might regret that when I got finished, but for now the camera was rolling. Jenny introduced me, and I started.

"As you know triage comes from a Latin origin and means to sort. Most of the time, you folks do a great job with that. However, in the short time I have been here, I have noted two areas that could use some improvement. The first area goes back to something that your mother might have said. 'Always wear clean underwear, you never know if you will be in an accident.' So, my challenge to you is this, in support of mothers everywhere we need to document the condition of the underwear of every patient who gets in an accident. We do mothers a great disservice when we don't check and document."

At first, there was an eerie silence, followed by cacophonous laughter.

"I recommend the CC, CS, SM, and FOS method of documentation."

There were giggles and cat calls. Jenny's face was red, and Mr. G was worried that he was going to dry off for a change. But undaunted, I continued. I had slides of old underwear that I had doctored up with brown shoe polish to make my in-service even more life-like.

"CC means completely clean. This would be a rare finding. CS means a couple stains. You have the option to include a number. Such as CS 3. SM means skid marks. Again, you have the option to include a number. Such as SM 1. You all know what FOS is, no number is needed."

They were rolling in the aisles, and Jenny was belly-laughing. I allowed a few minutes for the crowd to settle then I continued.

"The second area of triage that is important is room assignment. Why put a female pelvic problem in a room without a gynecologic table. It's inefficient and slows us down."

A hand went up, and I acknowledged it. "Yes, a question?"

It was from Dawn, one of the older and more experienced nurses. "How often does this occur? In my experience, pelvic problems are always put in the appropriate room."

"It happens all the time," I said. "In fact, I have two charts from the last week that show how serious the problem is. Dawn, unfortunately, one of the charts is yours."

She shot me an incredulous look as I put the slide of the chart on the screen.

The chief complaint read: "Laceration repaired last week, now has pussy discharge." The second one read: "Large mass on buttocks leaking pussy discharge."

Some nurses had a habit of using the word pussy to mean exuding pus, instead of the medical word, "purulent". This in-service would help end that practice.

I said, "Clearly, both patients required an exam of their pussy discharge. Now that is not a proper medical word, but we all know what a pussy is, don't we?"

This was met with whistles and catcalls, and Jenny rushing to shut off the recorder. I ended the session with some sage words of advice after posing a question.

"What two things should you never do in a bar?"

There were a few lewd answers screamed out, but I waved them off.

"First, you never mind your own business. Almost every night we get people in here who are injured in bar fights. What do most of them say? They say, 'I was just sitting there minding my own business when that bastard sucker punched me.' So, minding your own business can be dangerous in a bar. The second thing you never do is have two beers. You can have one, or three, or fifty, but never two. Why is that? Well almost every drunk we get in here who has caused a wreck claims to only have had two beers. So, there must something bad about that."

More laughs and whistles. I took a bow, and I thanked everyone for their attention. I further assured them that they would be even more valuable assets to the department with their added knowledge. The night staff filed out of the conference room to check the department and Jenny remained behind.

"I hope you're not too mad," I said sheepishly.

"How could I be mad? I'm an ER nurse and like our medics and doctors we live in the sewer. Nice in-service!!" Then she laughed so hard I thought she was going to pass out.

"Jenny, would you like to see a racehorse get born?"

"Wow," she said, "that would be awesome."

"You can also meet my mother and sister."

She laughed, "Pretty serious shit. When?"

"Tomorrow night, are you up for this? "

"No guts, no glory."

"Good I will send a car for you. I have to be at the track before you need to be picked up, but I will see you later. Be ready at 6 PM and make sure your underwear is clean."

She rolled her eyes. Before I could say anything else I heard Dawn scream "peds arrest" from triage. Jenny and I ran to the main resuscitation room as Dawn ran in with a blue toddler. The kid looked dead, but we still had to try to see what we could do.

A frantic set of parents burst into the room and proclaimed through sobs, "We went to check on her and found the sliding glass door open. We found her at the bottom of the pool. Save our baby, save our baby!" They screamed and cried.

Jenny went over to escort them to the family room to wait, but I shook my head no. I usually allowed parents to be present during a resuscitation. There were many studies that showed it was therapeutic for them to see that all was done to save their child. This didn't look like it would end well, and I thought they deserved to see that we gave her every chance. Jenny moved them to the side of the room and instructed one of the aides to sit with them.

No one could get an IV. After I got a tube in to breathe for the child, and made sure we tried to warm her, I knew I had to get IV access. The kid was cold and in shock. She was flatline on the monitor. I elected to insert an interosseous catheter. We had a nice device that drilled into the bone marrow of the child's lower leg. It was fairly easy and allowed for rapid vascular access in the event no one could get an IV. In less than one minute, it was in.

Dawn looked up, "How about a dose of EPI?"

"Good idea, please get the correct dose from the Broselow tape."

No one who isn't a pediatrician can remember the dosages for toddler resuscitative medications. You just don't use them often enough. Thank God. To help with the correct dosages, we used a tape that you placed the child on. Based on the child's length, the tape approximated the weight and gave you the dosage for every resuscitation drug. Better than estimating. The tape had this kid weighing eighteen pounds.

Before Dawn could answer, someone handed her a syringe with epinephrine at the correct dose for an eighteen-pounder. I looked down at the most beautiful, unattractive person I had ever seen. She was short and morbidly obese. Her hair was disheveled, and her face was covered in pitting acne. Her ass was as wide as she was tall, but she had the drug I needed in the correct dosage. I would have kissed her anywhere she wanted.

I have just met Crystal Francis PharmD. I remember reading somewhere that most resuscitations had better outcomes if a pharmacist was part of the team. Now I knew why. I winked at her. She had heard the call for a peds arrest in ED and she volunteered to help.

A couple rounds of resuscitation drugs later, a rapid heartbeat appeared on the screen. This was followed by Dawn screaming.

"I got a pulse!!!"

Before I knew what happened the parents were at the bedside. The blue toddler was now pink and fighting like hell to remove my tube. I asked for a versed drip, and Crystal had it ready in less than a minute. Now sedated, the child's heart rate decreased, and the BP continued to rise.

I put my arms around Mom and Dad, and we all thanked God.

I whispered to them. "We still don't know if her brain was damaged by the episode. We won't know that until she is evaluated at Children's Hospital, and eventually woken up. But so far, there is no reason to believe she doesn't have a chance to be ok."

I passed Dawn on the way out of the room. All she said was, "I am now a SM-1."

I replied. "Good for you, I know I am FOS."

We both grinned.

After the helicopter evacuated the child to Children's, the rest of the night was uneventful. Amos made a nice score on the asshole of the night. He chose the first patient and that was the winner. It's a big risk taking the first patient, but he made it work. After a peds arrest, no one usually wants to make a new bet. The complaint he picked looked innocent enough: "snake bite." The medic suspected that there was more to the story, and he was right.

The guy was drunk and had been cutting wood with a friend while drinking Fireball shots. Yep, they were using a chainsaw. Now, they didn't kill themselves with the chainsaw by some stroke of luck, but they pushed their good fortunes too far when they saw a snake. These Einsteins decided to catch it. OOPS, too bad you're sad, but this was a timber rattler, and it was poisonous. Our contestant got bit twice. One call to Crystal and the antivenom arrived in the correct dosage. Now to get this asshole a brain transplant. That will take some doing. Nothing else came close and Amos won the cash. When the sun rose, we all wandered home, and wondered how our little girl was doing.

I called PC on the way home.

"Why the hell are you waking me up?"

He was ticked off that I woke him up, but he got over it when I pitched my deal.

"Can you take the night off from the track tomorrow and pick up a friend and take her to the clubhouse?"

"ZZ trying to get laid? This sounds like a Mr. G project to me."

"Something like that."

He knew the rest of the drill. He would entertain her while I was racing. After I finished my last race, he would bring her to the barn to meet Mom and Stephanie. He agreed.

"I have a few bets for you to place."

He really liked the sound of that.

CHAPTER 14

Fired Up Farms
Krenshaw, NJ
1500 July 1

I made a brief stop at the track to train just one horse and I headed home. I was asleep by 9 AM. I was startled by the phone ringing at 3 PM. It was Marie, the school nurse, and she was terrified.

"Hello, I'll be right there." I screamed to Stephanie. "Tell Mom I went over to the school. One of the kids is sick."

"OK"

I ran over to the school. I arrived in the infirmary short of breath. A seven-year-old was lying on the cot. He was breathing rapidly. More rapidly than me and he appeared to be unconscious. I did a sternal rub to no avail. The nurse had checked blood sugar, and it was normal. Marie helped me remove his clothes, and I froze. I had only seen it once before in my life, meningococcemia. The rash was red speckles, but they would not blanche with pressure. Marie said the kid was fine this AM. Now he was near death.

I turned to see Stephanie enter the room.

"Stephanie, call 911 and request a medical helicopter to this location. The destination will be Children's Hospital. Diagnosis meningococcemia, suspect meningococcal meningitis."

"ZZ, fucking speak English!"

"Sorry Stephanie, just request a helicopter come here to take a child to Children's. I will call them with an update when I can."

Marie started an IV and I did a quick exam of the child's neck. It was stiff as a board. Shit, shit. Meningitis caused by meningococcemia.

This kid could be dead by sunset. I knew I had to get some antibiotics into him, but we didn't carry any intravenous antibiotics for kids. Then I remembered that we did have IV antibiotics for the horses. But which of those were safe for kids and would take care of meningococcemia?

I speed-dialed Crystal Francis, the pharmacist. I had put her number in my contact list after she helped us so much last night. She answered on the second ring.

"Crystal this is Dr. Zander, I need your help fast."

"Where are you? In the ER?"

"No, I am at the Always Hope School. It's a school for special needs kids, and I've got a kid with an incredibly special need."

"I will help however I can."

"I have a seven-year-old with probable meningococcal meningitis, I am evacuating him to Children's. He is moribund and I want to get some antibiotics into him stat. I only have vet drugs in my location. Can you help me?"

"Call you in five or less."

As I waited for her call, I dialed Children's and got a referral specialist. He agreed to accept the transfer and asked to transfer me to one of the PICU (Pediatric Intensive Care Unit) attendings.

"This is Dr Early," a squeaky voice stated. "What do you have?"

I gave her a brief rundown and told her. "I might have some antibiotics to give."

"If you know it is safe, please give the antibiotics as soon as possible. They are critical. You wouldn't happen to have a spinal tap tray available? We could save some valuable time here if you do. The cultures are infinitely better if they are obtained before any antibiotic administration."

The helicopter wouldn't arrive for at least thirty minutes. Marie looked for the kit we needed to do a lumbar puncture, while I took an incoming call from Crystal.

"OK Dr. Zander. I found a website that crisscrosses drugs that can be used in animals and humans. Do you have any Zestend?"

"No," I said.

"How about Frutomal, or Drastican? "

"Drastican we have."

"Great. What is your child's weight?"

"About 25 kg."

She paused for a minute, and I heard a few keystrokes. "Give him 400 milligrams of Drastican IV. It comes in 1000 mg vials."

"Thanks Crystal, I owe you again."

I hung up. Stephanie ran to the barn to get the Drastican. It was in a refrigerator in the tack room. The nurse found an old spinal tap kit. It was expired for use, but that only had to do with its sterility. I cracked it open. Any port in a storm.

I finally wised up and had a mask placed on the child, and on the nurse, and I. His secretions were highly contagious. Why didn't I think of this earlier? We got the kid on his side, and I positioned him as best I could for the tap. I felt for his posterior spinous processes and then I found the top of his pelvis. The space I wanted to enter was in the midline. I went back to feel the spine and then I painted his back with betadine. I knew it had to dry to be effective but, I had no time to waste. I draped his back and proceeded as Stephanie arrived.

"I need 400 mg."

I had taught her how to get antibiotics ready for the horses, but I would double-check this special dose.

"Stephanie please put on a mask."

I made my first pass with the needle. The kid moved some, which was a good sign that his brain was still somewhat alive. I repositioned him and went in again. This time I felt the slight pop that I was hoping to feel. I held the device and carefully removed the hub. Thick white pus dripped from the needle. Spinal fluid was supposed to be clear and colorless. This was the worst fluid I had ever seen.

I collected my samples and removed the device. Stephanie handed the antibiotic to the nurse after I double-checked the dose. I opened the emergency kit and prepared to intubate the child. As the tube slipped in, he coughed. A large chunk of mucous hit my protective visor. Thank God I remembered to put it on. I heard an ambulance approaching to establish a landing zone, followed by a helicopter.

The child was carefully packaged and whisked to the chopper. In less than twenty minutes, he would be in his PICU bed. I needed to get to the track when Crystal called back.

"What are you doing about prophylaxis?" she asked.

What was I doing about prophylaxis? Shit, I totally forgot. I and the nurse had definitely been exposed. Stephanie was in the room when we did the resuscitation and procedures. Who else had the child come in contact with? Meningococcus was a nasty and contagious bug. I needed to stay here and manage this, or others could die.

As all of this ran through my head, Crystal asked, "Can I help?"

I hated to ask her, but I needed to get to the track, and I had no other option.

"As I told you, I am at the Always Hope School. We have about thirty kids and one hundred staff. I have no idea who may have been exposed. I have a number of races at the track tonight, but the kids and staff are more important."

"Dr. Zander I have a brother with special needs. I know all about the school and I would love to help. I can come right over and assess the situation. Because it is an emergency my license permits me to prescribe in this case. I can manage the situation, and it would be my honor if you would permit me."

Wow, she was beautiful. I also knew that the nursing staff and therapists would give her any assistance she needed.

"I will be forever indebted to you."

"You'll get my bill," she giggled and then she added. "Besides yourself, was there anyone else exposed to the child who won't be there when I arrive?"

"Just Stephanie and I." She arranged for some rifampin for me and Stephanie.

CHAPTER 15

Racetrack Road

Krenshaw, NJ

1730 July 1

I called PC and asked him to stop at the pharmacy to get the prescription. Mom had packed food to go. Stephanie and I took off for the track. Mom would come later in her truck.

I asked Stephanie, "Could you be pregnant?"

She got super pissed and her face turned purple.

"I never fucked. I never fucked. Ok once, but I didn't like it. Months ago, so I am not in foal."

"OK Stephanie, maybe a little too much information. I just had to ask because of the medicine I need to give you."

"Oh," she said.

"It will make your piss bright yellow," I added.

Stephanie looked at the floor without speaking. I continued in silence as I pondered who her partner had been.

PC stopped at the pharmacy before picking up Jenny. PC walked slowly up to her apartment door and expected to wait. He knocked and the door opened immediately. She was ready, right-on time. And boy was she ever ready. She had on the tightest white pants that PC had ever seen. Not tight because she was fat. Tight in that they hugged her very attractive pelvic features. Her auburn hair was sparkling in the sun. She flashed him a big smile with her perfect white teeth outlined by pouty lips and bright red cheeks. She was glowing hot, and she knew it.

"Hi, I'm Johnson Stevens," PC said as he stretched out his hand.

"I was expecting Pisscatcher," said Jenny with a slight grin.

"Well, that's also my name, especially at the track."

Jenny asked "Where are we going? I was invited to watch a racehorse get born. This must be an induction or a c-section because ZZ seemed to know it would be tonight. These things can't exactly be planned."

"Well, you don't know ZZ very well. He plans more shit than anyone I know."

Jenny chewed on that a second and asked, "Do you know about any old girlfriends ZZ had?"

"A little above my pay grade, sweetie. I only see him at the track and occasionally at his farm. I haven't seen him for a week."

"Why the name Pisscatcher?" Jenny asked with a raised, but beautifully made-up eyebrow.

"I catch piss."

"So do I, but that is for samples in the ER. Most of the time I use a catheter."

"I use a cup on the end of a stick. Safer than trying to stick a catheter in the bladder of a thousand-pound beast. The winner of a race, and as many horses that the judges want samples from, are kept after the race until they urinate. When they start to go, I get my cup on a stick and catch my sample. I label it and send it off to the state lab."

"Your job sounds a lot like mine," laughed Jenny.

"I also am a CPA. Trust me, catching piss is more exciting."

They arrived at the track and Jenny looked surprised.

"They deliver baby horses at the track?"

"Who said anything about delivering baby horses?" chuckled PC.

He got a kick out of the fact that I had kept her in the dark. They entered the track and took the elevator to the top of the clubhouse. They proceeded to the "Millions Club" which was a club restricted to owners and guests of owners. PC showed his and Jenny's identification to the guard at the door, and they were permitted entry.

The Millions Club was extravagant. Perfectly set tables with live flowers and small television monitors filled the room. Beautiful pictures of racehorses and famous races covered most of the walls. The front of the room was all glass. It overlooked the racetrack. They were escorted to their table by a hostess dressed as a cowgirl. Their table was right at the window and was adorned with a beautiful bouquet of roses. Tied to the bouquet was a carrot. A note was attached to the carrot with Jenny's name on it. She opened it.

"Sorry for being so cryptic. I hope you enjoy tonight. I will see you in the barn after the races. You can give the carrot to one of the horses, unless someone slips in the club, and it disappears. Ha ha, ZZ."

They ordered drinks and PC remembered that he needed to get the prescription to me. He showed the medicine to Jenny.

"What's this stuff for?"

"Rifampin, it's an antibiotic But I never see it used much. Makes your urine very yellow."

"Well, he and his sister have to take this for some reason."

"I don't know anything about it."

PC got Jenny a racing program. She read through it while PC went over to the paddock to deliver the medicine. There was an article about me returning to the track. There were pictures of me in my younger days, and pictures of me with Mom and a very pretty blonde. Jenny was happy to read that it was my sister Stephanie.

She didn't know how to read the racing lines, but she picked through each race and noted that I was driving in the first four races. Three of the horses were owned by the Fired Up Farms and the last was not. Jenny also noted that Billie "Cha-ching" Browner was the leading driver at the track. He was in almost every race. Every time he was driving for Supreme Stables. They were by far the leading barn at the track.

PC got back and handed Jenny a headset. He also had one.

"This is something new at the track. Trying to catch up with NASCAR, I guess. We will be able to hear from ZZ during the race. We can't talk to him, but we can hear what he has to say about the race."

He explained about the races and briefly about betting. He told her that he would be able to watch most of the races with her, but he would be busy betting right up until the race started.

"Do you have a gambling problem that I should call the 800 number for?"

He laughed and said, "No, not as long as I win."

They finished their dinner and ordered some coffee. The bugle sounded and the horses came on to the track for the first race. I was driving the eight horse, Supreme Taco. She was a gray horse and stood out like a sore thumb in the post-parade. I was adorned in my racing colors, white pants with a white jacket with gold stripes down the sleeves. On my back were two large gold Zs. They had flames on them that made them look like they were moving and moving fast. I had on a gold helmet that was complimented by gold reflective sunglasses. The announcer said that Supreme Taco was owned by the Fired Up Farm.

Jenny asked, "Why is she was not named Fired Up Taco, or something like that?"

"Stephanie claimed her from Supreme stables a month ago for $50,000. She had been sold for $800,000 as a yearling. To this point she had raced ten times as a two-year-old and thirteen times as a three-year-old, and never got close to winning a race. This year she is four years old. So far this year she has raced seven times and finished last six out of the seven times. The only reason Stephanie bought her was for breeding. She is a dismal racehorse."

They were interrupted by ZZ speaking, "Hello Jenny, hi PC, thanks for the meds. Had a kid with meningococcemia at the school. Stephanie and I are taking the medication for prophylaxis. I don't want you to think I have the cooties. Enjoy the races. See you in the barn. ZZ out."

PC explained further that there was a chance that this horse might race a little better. ZZ's mother had a formula for horses they bought that had not been racing well. It started with a complete head-to-toe vet exam. That included x-rays and ultrasounds. Any injuries were diagnosed, and a treatment plan was started. The horse was then tube wormed. They use NG tubes like you do in the ER. They use them to administer a worming medicine that is much stronger than the ones usually used.

This was followed by two weeks in the field to run, play, and be a horse again. If they had wounds that needed attention, they got it right in the field. At some point they got their teeth evaluated by an equine dentist. A lot of these horses had sore mouths from bad or neglected teeth. The week before they returned to the races, they were jogged daily and returned to the field. No fast miles, just light jogging. Sometimes, these overpriced horses were overtrained. People who had paid too much wanted big returns on their investments. Often, they pushed them too hard and ignored the little things like worming and mouth care. Many of these horses were worn down and tired of being abused. It was amazing how much good could happen in three short weeks.

At two minutes to post, PC excused himself and went to the betting window. Supreme Taco was 18 to 1 odds. But when the horses lined up behind the starting gate, she had dropped to 7 to 1. PC returned to the table with a fistful of tickets.

"What did you bet?" Jenny wanted to know.

PC said nothing and motioned for her to watch out the window. He offered her some binoculars and adjusted the table television monitor so she could see the race on there too.

The track announcer took over. "They round the turn and here they come for the start of tonight's racing program," he bellowed.

Over the headset, Jenny heard a lot of hoofbeats and some talking and whistling. It was just the drivers getting ready for the start. The car and attached starting gate pulled away as it crossed the start line, and the race began.

The announcer made the call. "That's Big Runner leaving from the inside, Hapenstance breaking sharply from the five-hole, but the fastest of all is Supreme Taco going right to the front."

Just then, Big Runner, driven by Billie "Cha-ching" pulled to the outside to pass Supreme Taco.

PC screamed, "Park his stuttering ass out."

In her headset, Jenny heard me say, "Fuck you Ba-Ba-Ba-Ba-Billie, you ain't getting the front!"

"We-we-we-we will see," replied Billie as he whacked his horse with the whip.

The announcer called it. "That's Big Runner making a move to the front, but ZZ says *no way today* and drives on. They pass the quarter in 27.2. Supreme Taco and Big Runner are throwing down right here and now. Billie "Cha-Ching" urges Big Runner on, but he cannot clear to the top. They reached the half in a blistering 55 seconds."

Jenny heard me again in her headset. "Ha ha, how do-do you like like it out-out there Billie?"

That was followed by another chorus of badly stuttered "fuck yous" from Billie.

Jenny also noted that Billie was driving his horse furiously but I just kind of sat there.

She asked PC, "Why is ZZ stuttering?"

"Billie stutters a ton. ZZ is just doing it to piss him off, get him off his game. Seems to be working."

In the next instant, she heard me whistle to Supreme Taco. Then she heard me say, "Time for you to become a racehorse."

The announcer crooned. "ZZ pops the plugs. Supreme Taco seems to be full of hot sauce tonight. She leaves Big Runner in her dust."

PC interrupted the announcer to tell Jenny that she was seeing a racehorse get born. With every step, this mare was forgetting how much she had been abused and beaten, and how much she hated racing. She recognized some soft hands and a caring tone from her driver. She felt good racing. She was in no pain, and she loved what she was doing. Right now, thirty-two pairs of chromosomes were unfolding. The monster racehorse she was bred to be, was emerging.

"Supreme Taco opens a five-length lead on the field. She is going smooth and easy, maybe tonight she will get that first elusive win. The third quarter was in 27 seconds"!!! The announcer was getting hoarse.

I had a ton of horse in front of me and I knew it. I screamed to her, "Get ready for the Army."

Supreme Taco rounded the last turn and entered the top of the stretch. And there they were, about twenty autistic kids and their handlers. They were all at the rail screaming. Plus, they were rolling their right arms back like a third base coach does when he wants the runner to go for the plate. Supreme Taco had a blind on her left eye but none on the right, by plan. She saw the crowd rolling their arms and she dug in.

The announcer hit a higher octave and screamed, "Supreme Taco shows her heels to the field. Final quarter in 27.4, mile in 1:49.4 Wow, she really made her first win something else!!!"

PC grabbed Jenny's hand, and they caught the elevator to ground level.

"Where are we going?" asked Jenny.

"To get your picture taken sweetie," laughed PC.

CHAPTER 16

They exited the elevator and made their way to the winner's circle. There, they met Damian and his therapist. He was the chosen child to get to the winner's circle. It was way too difficult and time-consuming to get all twenty kids there, so they took turns.

Stephanie had jumped on my bike and rode back with me to the winner's circle. She jumped off the side of the bike and held Taco for the picture as everyone crowded around.

"What did you think of the birth?" I asked Jenny laughingly.

"Not what I expected but pretty cool."

"Did you like your flowers and carrot?"

"Flowers yes, carrot no."

I whispered in her ear, "Do you have on clean underwear?"

"No, I'm not wearing any." Jenny replied with a big grin.

That made sense. Those pants were way too tight to permit anything else to be worn.

Back in the clubhouse, PC went to cash the tickets. He came back with a fistful of $100 bills and gave two to Jenny.

"What's this for?"

"ZZ asked me to bet $20 to win on her for you. Your ticket was worth $200."

"I can't take that," Jenny stammered.

"Sure, you can. You can bet it on ZZ. You may also want to come back and bet on Taco for about the next five to six weeks in a row. She will be in cheap and will murder them for a while. With what you have left over you can buy some underwear. People not wearing underwear are either very poor, or very confident, or both."

PC laughed as Jenny's face turned red.

I was driving Hubba Hubba in the second race for trainer Bill Mallory.

"In the big scheme of things Hubba is not a great horse. In fact, if ZZ hadn't raced him well in that qualifier a few weeks ago, he would probably have been sold for meat," explained PC.

"You have to be kidding, meat?"

"That's an area of the racing business that no one likes to discuss. But your boyfriend spared him from that outcome, at least temporarily."

Jenny was shocked, but it was clear that PC wanted to change the subject. "You know that ZZ is racing to make money to save the farm?"

"Yes, he told me. Can he make much money doing this?"

PC went on to explain. "ZZ makes 5% of what the horse makes. The purse in this race is $6,000. With a win the owner gets $3000, and ZZ gets $150."

"That's all??" she asked.

"Yeah, he is taking all comers and trying to get himself back into racing shape. In order to drive good horses, you have to drive a few that are less than stellar. But if this was a $100,000 race and his horse won, he would get $2500 for less than two minutes work."

"Now that can add up." Jenny acknowledged.

I said nothing as I scored Hubba Hubba down. All that Jenny and PC heard was hoofbeats until they lined up behind the gate. Hubba Hubba had the four-hole. In the five-hole was Supreme Actor driven by Billie. Billie came out with a relatively stutter-free sentence.

"Hey-hey twit, don't get in my waw-a way."

I looked over and laughed, "You-you-you goin' down man."

The track announcer again took over. "They are off. Supreme Actor to the top followed by Hubba Hubba."

We got to the quarter in a slow 29 seconds. To this point, it was an unexciting race. Then the announcer woke back up.

"Five Under Par pulls from the three-hole and tries to get to the front. He is gaining steadily first over but just can't clear Supreme Actor. Billie 'Cha-ching' is sitting chilly in the bike and parks Five Under Par out. But Five Under Par isn't ready to concede. They race neck and neck down the backside. They reach the three-quarter pole in 1:30 but Five Under Par is fading, I guess that's better than hooking," quipped the announcer.

Five Under Par fell back around the turn and I pulled Hubba Hubba to the outside. He was surprisingly live.

The announcer jumped back in and screamed. "Here comes ZZ and Hubba Hubba, going right on by. Hubba Hubba gets to go somewhere he's never been, to the winner's circle. Mile in 1:58. First career victory for Hubba Hubba. ZZ has taken two horses to the promised land tonight."

PC cashed another sheaf of tickets and ordered more drinks. Up in the third race was Fired Up Jackie. Jenny noticed that she was the favorite to win a sire's stake race.

"What is a sire's stake race?" she asked.

PC gave her an abbreviated answer. "All of the horses in this race were bred to sires who stand in NJ. The owners must make sustaining payments at certain times in the horse's life to keep them eligible. The ones that look like they may be able to win are entered in the race. The purse is $150,000 so a win means $75,000 for Fired Up Farms."

ZZ was totally silent. PC went to bet and came back.

"What did you bet?" Jenny asked.

"Nothing, I wanted to bet Fired Up Jackie. But her odds are so low that it wasn't worth it. I like her a lot, but Supreme Firepower looks like she could give ZZ some trouble."

Jenny said, "What the hell is that in my ear?"

"That would be ZZ singing but I can't make out the words."

"It sounds like Stone in Love by Journey," said Jenny.

"OMG," said PC, "I can't believe he is Stone in Loving you on the first track date. He never does that."

Jenny had no idea what that meant but she did know that she was hearing some of the worst singing she had ever heard. Fortunately, the singing was somewhat drowned out when the announcer started.

"They are off. Supreme Firepower jumps smartly to the front. Supreme Slapshot gets away second. Great Karma trots third. Amen Brother is caught on the outside praying for a hole to open. Freestone Peach is fifth, XXX Rated is sixth, Uganda Mamma is seventh and Fired Up Jackie can see them all."

PC was reading the next race in the program and Jenny asked why he wasn't watching the race. "Tell me if something happens," he said without taking his eyes off the program.

"Like what?"

"You'll know." That's all he said, and he returned to the program.

The announcer was very animated. "Supreme Firepower takes them to the half in a leisurely 58.4. Supreme Slapshot is right on her heels. Out of the five-hole pops Freestone Peach first over. Fired up Jackie is anything but fired up. She can still see them all from dead last."

As they rounded the turn past the half-mile pole Jenny screamed at PC.

"He is still singing terribly, but he is moving all around in the sulky. He looks like he is trying to start a lawnmower." PC jumped up with the glasses and screamed.

"I hope he does that one more time."

"What is he doing?" Jenny asked.

"He has these delusions that he is starting up a jet engine, like you would a lawnmower. He starts one on each side and he is off. He only does that if he is sitting on a ton of horse. Grab your ass because this might get interesting."

I yelled "fire" and popped Jackie to the outside. The announcer saw it unfolding and screamed "and here comes Fired Up Jackie, now 7th, now 6th, now 5th, now 4th, now 3rd."

Jackie rolled past those horses like they were standing still. At the last second, Russell Flannigan pulled Supreme Slapshot out of the two-hole. Clearly, that was an attempt to block me from swooping to the front. As Russel did that, Billie let his horse loose and opened a two-length lead. I jerked Jackie to the pylons and left a surprised Russell Flanigan, sucking air on the outside. I flipped him off using my right hand.

I quickly caught up to Supreme Firepower. I got so close that Jackie was banging on Billie's helmet with her nose. We rounded the final turn, and The Army was on their feet.

Jenny wanted to know, "What are they doing this time?"

They were waving one arm up and down. PC looked and said, "They are striking a hammer. They want ZZ to put the hammer down and end this race."

I pulled to the outside and let Jackie trot on. She quickly pulled beside Firepower. I then made a motion with my left arm like I was striking a nail with a hammer. I gave Jackie her marching orders and she took off. The Army erupted in screams.

I flipped Billie off with my left hand as the announcer proclaimed, "Much to the delight of the Awesome Army, ZZ puts the hammer down and gives Cha-ching that famous Zander salute. Fired Up Jackie pulls away to win by seven lengths. From dead last to first. This is one very serious filly."

PC heard me talking to the outrider. "Jet engines I tell you, jet engines!!"

I got Jackie back to the winner's circle and this time I had Jenny sit on the sulky. I gave her a nice pinch on the ass and told PC, "My horse in the next race is scratched. You can come to the barn now."

CHAPTER 17

Barn 14

Miracle Mile Racetrack and Casino

Krenshaw, NJ

2200 July 1

There was no celebrating going on in barn 14.

"What the fuck is the matter with you Billie?" screamed Deuce. "I lost my ass tonight, particularly on Firepower. I swear I will start to use The Blue Man (nickname for Nick Demary) to drive. He isn't flashy, but he doesn't fuck up as much as you do."

"Sorry Mr. Ho-Ho Hofecker," stammered Billie without looking up. He had been studying his boots since Deuce began his berating.

"First of all, they stole that mare Taco off us for $50,000. We paid $800,000! You were the last of three drivers to work with her. Zander does in a month what you shitheads couldn't do in a year. I am not putting up with this crap. Do you understand?"

"Ya-ya-ya sir-sir-sir, I do. This is r-r-r-r-r-r racing. There are ga-ga-ga good nights and ba-ba-ba bad, and this was a bad n-n-n-n-n-n night."

"You have no idea how bad a night you will have if this doesn't turn around. The Millions Mile is just around the corner. Get your head out of your ass."

Deuce stormed off as Billie stuttered under his breath.

On the way back to the hospital, Deuce made a phone call, but he got only voicemail. He left a short message. He hung up as he arrived back at the hospital. He parked in his reserved spot and made his way to the employee entrance. He turned left and walked past an empty conference room. Then, he accessed a security camera on his phone and ascertained that no one could see him. He unlocked the door in the hallway marked "electrical panels" and closed the door behind him. He located the keypad on the far right and entered a fifteen-digit code. One of the sidewalls retracted. He quickly entered an anteroom as the wall slid back into position. He put his thumb on the fingerprint reader and then peered into the iris scanner. The final door opened. He entered a large lounge area with banks of computers and screens. He was greeted by Kris (Knuckles) Markovich.

"Tom, how the hell are you, kill them at the races?"

"Unfortunately, my driver had his head up his ass and I lost mine," said Deuce as he shook his head in disgust.

"Well, this might put a smile on your face. Got a three-mil contract tonight. NFL QB, two-time loser with his third positive on the way to the lab."

"Now that does take the sting and stink out of a bad evening," Deuce said as he poured himself a generous drink of scotch.

"The details are on the computer. Is there anything I can do before I leave? I got a first-rate hooker stopping by my apartment in a half hour."

"Nah Kris, I 'm fine. Go get your rocks off."

Barn 7

2230

After clearing security, PC showed Jenny into the barn. She saw a long line of stalls with a trunk in front of each stall. The ground was perfectly raked and cleaner than most restaurants. He quickly found Mom and introduced her to Jenny. They chit-chatted for a few minutes, then I arrived with Fired Up Jackie and Stephanie. I jumped off, unhooked the bike, and removed the equipment. I helped put two blankets on Jackie. Stephanie started to walk her in slow circles in front of the barn.

I asked, "Who needs a beer?"

Jenny, PC, and I opened our beers. Stephanie opted for a flavored iced tea. Mom went down barn row checking on horses. We stood at the door of the barn and watched Stephanie cool out Jackie.

"Stephanie, I want you to meet Jenny," I said.

"Hi Jenny, are you porking ZZ?" Stephanie asked with a very serious look on her face.

I screamed, "Stephanie, you promised!"

"Sorry, nice to meet you, Jenny."

Jenny was red-faced and looked like she wanted to be someplace else. PC lightened the mood when he talked about my singing. He knew Stephanie and was used to helping defuse these moments.

"Your singing is below bad, but your driving makes up for it."

He handed me a wad of cash. I counted out $1,000 and handed that back to him.

"Another 200 nights like this and we will be out of debt." I laughed as I finished my beer. "But it's a start. PC, I'll drive Jenny home."

"Great, I have an early audit tomorrow anyway. Good night."

Mom spoke up. "I'll wait for Stephanie to cool out Jackie."

"What time should we expect you home ZZ?" Stephanie asked.

Now here I am almost thirty. I really wanted to go to Jenny's and maybe spend the night. But my little sister was raining on my parade.

"Probably two or three Stephanie," I said.

"Don't be late," she laughed.

Jenny and I discussed the races on the way home.

"What did you do to Taco to make her improve so much?" she asked.

"Rest, worming, dentist etc. There were a lot of things."

"Which is the most important? Can you do that with all horses?"

She almost seemed a little too interested. She wanted details about things that should have been a little beyond her limited knowledge of racing. Alarm bells were going off in my head. But in my pants, Mr. G told me to pay it no mind, and I obliged. I got back to the farm at 3 AM with a smile on my face.

CHAPTER 18

Emergency Department
Supreme Medical Center
0050 July 13

The weeks quickly passed. Fired Up Rio won her second start, but each race brought out another quirk of hers that needed to be resolved. Stephanie repeatedly changed equipment. Every now and again, I had to use the whip, which I hated. I knew Rio had tremendous potential, but she was somewhat of a head case. The rest of her races for this year were stakes caliber. She would have to get better to keep on winning.

Tonight, I used my card to enter the employee entrance. I was late because the weather was terrible. It was pouring down sheets of rain. There was a thick, pea soup fog. I was hoping to avoid a lecture by Jenny for being late. I was surprised when I was greeted by a smiling Jenny who told me things were quiet.

"Way to go Jenny, you asshole," I bellowed.

Everyone in the ER knew that if anyone mentioned that it was quiet, when it was quiet, then all hell would soon break loose. The nurse manager just jinxed us! No sooner had I donned my white coat and poured a cup of coffee when the radio came to life.

"Supreme Medical, Supreme Medical, this is medic unit 46."

It sounded like Amos, but he sounded harried. That was a problem. Most medics see enough blood and gore that they never get excited. When they do get excited, it means that you were about to have a bad night.

He continued, "We are in route to a two-car MVA with one known fatality and a pregnant woman entrapped." Nothing gets medics more wound up than a pregnant patient.

"This is med com physician 2436. Medic unit 46, I recommend helicopter standby for immediate evacuation of the patient to a trauma center once extricated."

"Med com physician 2436 from medic unit 46, helicopter evac not possible due to weather. All patients will be transferred to your facility."

"Copy that medic unit 46. We will be awaiting your arrival and standing by for anything further you might need. Med com physician 2436, Supreme Medical, out."

"Who is on call for Obstetrics?" I asked as I tried to get my head around what was unfolding.

"Dr. Hyman," replied Anita, the ward secretary.

"You have got to be shitting me, an OB guy named Hyman? What's his first name, Buster?" It was now.

Anita blushed as Jenny quickly volunteered, "Dr. Hyman is an older physician. In fact, he delivered me!"

"Get him in here now!" I screamed as the radio began to squawk again.

"Medic unit 46 to med com 2436: we are on scene. Pick-up truck t-boned a Prius. Prius was pushed into a bridge abutment. Truck rolled over multiple times. Driver of the Prius is dead, front seat passenger is entrapped. She is unconscious, Glasgow three, Cheyne Stokes respirations. Her skull is open, and brain matter is protruding from her ear. She appears to be near-term in her pregnancy. I cannot access her to evaluate the uterus."

"Medic 46, this is med com 2436. Whenever possible, intubate the victim. You may need to try it with her still in the car. Do it orally, as she likely has facial fractures, and a nasal approach isn't wise. If the baby is still viable, we need to protect the mother's airway and keep her pressure up. It doesn't sound like the mother is viable. But if we can get her here, we might be able to save the baby."

"Copy that med com 2436, will supplement with 100% oxygen, attempt an IV and oral intubation," replied Amos.

"Med Com 2436, this is Medic 21. I have the driver of the pick-up truck. He is also unconscious with a Glasgow coma score of seven. He has extremely labored breathing, no breath sounds on the right, and his trachea is deviated to the left. BP is 40 palp."

"Medic 21 from Med Com 2436. Sounds like a tension pneumothorax. Immediately needle decompress the right chest. I will standby."

Although only twenty seconds passed, it seemed like an eternity. Finally, the radio squawked again.

"Med Com 2436, this is Medic 21. Needle decompression done, a large rush of air. Respirations less labored, BP 80."

"Roger that medic 21. When possible, intubate the patient, start two large bore IVs with NSS wide open, and transport. If he develops more respiratory distress, decompress his chest again."

"Copy that, medic 21 out."

Jenny ran over and looked very harried as she relayed a message.

"Dr. Hyman called back. He recommends that the pregnant patient be taken directly to the trauma center. He does not feel it's appropriate for the patient to be brought here under any circumstance."

"Well fuck him, he's wrong. The patient is likely dead either way but the baby's only chance to survive might be an emergency C-section. Ground transport to the trauma center will add an additional forty-five minutes. The kid may not have that much time," I fumed.

"Med Com 2436 from medic 46."

"Go 46," I replied.

"Patient is intubated, two lines running, her abdomen is intermittently tense. I think she went into labor. No sign of vaginal bleeding. Bp 70/30, pupils fixed and dilated. Glasgow coma three. Dispatch has requested that we transport her directly to a trauma center on the advice of Dr. Hyman, who called them. Do you concur?"

"What is your ETA here, and to the trauma center?" I asked.

"Ten minutes to you. With current weather and reports of flooded roads, at least an hour to the trauma center."

"Medic 46, the patient is to be transported here. Prepare to perform CPR to support the fetus if the mother goes into cardiac arrest. If possible, place the patient on her left side."

"Copy that, Med Com. Medic 46 out."

"Call the surgeon on call, and Hyman. Ask them both to come to the ER stat," I screamed at Jenny. "Get a couple OB nurses down here. Ask them to bring an OR C-section pack with them. See if they can bring a bassinet with a warmer."

Jenny ran to the phone and made the calls.

I wanted to get both resuscitation rooms set up, but I was interrupted by a stroke alert call from the triage nurse. Forty-five-year-old male with sudden onset of right-sided weakness and speech difficulty. Shit! Shit! Damn that Jenny for saying how quiet it was. I met the stroke victim in room 12 and confirmed that the symptom onset was less than one hour. His physical exam confirmed a probable left middle cerebral artery stroke. I requested a stat CT scan and asked neurology to be stat paged.

Dr. Chew called back almost immediately. I gave him a brief report on the patient.

"Can you come in to manage this?" I begged. "I have two critically ill trauma patients in route."

"No problem, be there in less than ten minutes. Have the pharmacist prepare the TPA based upon our protocol. The TPA is NOT to be administered until I review the CT scan."

TPA is a very potent clot buster. It just might reverse this patient's stroke symptoms if given in time and under the right circumstances. It could also kill him if used inappropriately. I was happy to turn the case over to Dr. Chew. With what was coming my way I couldn't devote the time to the stroke patient that he needed. I knew he was in good hands.

Jenny met me as I exited the exam room and gave me some news that I didn't want to hear. "Dr. Hyman is refusing to come in. His opinion is that the patient should never be brought here. The surgeon called back, but he couldn't be here for an hour. He is at his cabin in the woods."

"Call a code violet," I screamed.

"You can't do that without speaking to the president of the medical staff, who happens to be Dr. Hyman," screamed back Jenny.

"Just fucking call it! I take full responsibility."

A code violet was a disaster call involving trauma. It required all available surgeons and ER physicians to report to the ER immediately. The bylaws were clear that anyone who was in town had to respond, or they would lose their privileges. It even further stipulated that any physician who felt that he/she was impaired at the time for any reason had to be driven to the hospital. Their being impaired was not an issue if they were not on call. But this rule had been put into place because many physicians in the past had claimed impairment to avoid responding to a code violet. Once evaluated, they would be excused from serving, but they had to respond. So much for the Hippocratic Oath.

CHAPTER 19

Emergency Department
Supreme Medical Center
0120 June 13

The first in the door was medic 21 with the driver of the truck. He was intubated but was still unconscious. Dr. Stanton was the first general surgeon to arrive. He went into the trauma room. Jenny drew some labs and labeled them. She used what we called a "John Doe" trauma pack, as we had not yet identified this victim. Once I made sure Dr. Stanton had all the help and equipment he needed, I exited the room. I almost ran straight into Deuce. He glared at me and asked where Dr. Hofecker was.

"How the hell should I know? He's off tonight." I shouted back.

Deuce put his head down and quietly said, "He was in the wreck. He was driving the truck." Before I could think, I put my arm around his shoulder.

"Mr. Hofecker, I'm so sorry. He's in room four. Dr. Stanton is with him now. I will have Jenny give you an update as soon as possible."

He was trembling and so was I. I walked him to a chair in the nurse's station and went back into the room to tell Jenny. Dr. Stanton placed a chest tube in Hofucker's right chest and got back a lot of air and blood. His blood pressure had risen to 90 and he was starting to buck the tube in his throat. The plan was to paralyze him to get him to CT. That would show what was up in his head, and further evaluate his chest and abdomen. Dr Stanton had ordered a catheter placed in Hofucker's bladder. I filled Jenny in as another nurse was cutting away his blood-soaked pants and underwear. She let out a terrified scream.

We all ran to her side, and then we all stopped. What we saw was the bloody stump of a completely amputated penis. I pulled Jenny and Dr. Stanton aside to inform them that their patient was Dr. Hofecker. I told them that Mr. Hofecker was sitting in the nurse's station. Jenny left with the blood samples. After she sent them on their way to the lab in the pneumatic tube, she sat with Mr. Hofecker.

The sound of another medic unit's siren drew closer. Within minutes, the door to the ambulance opened. The sight was not pretty. A formerly beautiful twenty-something blond was reduced to a bloody pulp of a head that was split open like a coconut. Brain matter was coming out of her ears along with blood and spinal fluid. Her blood pressure was 30. She was being ventilated with a bag-valve-mask, but her oxygen saturation was very low at eighty-five percent. I ordered some dopamine and asked one of the medics to start CPR until we got the pressure up. Crystal arrived and I took a deep breath. It was so good to see her in this situation. It helped me calm down.

The OB nurse finally got a monitor on the abdomen and the fetus was still alive. Unfortunately, the pattern on the monitor showed extreme fetal distress.

She screamed, "If we don't get this kid out of there in the next few minutes, it will die before the mother."

I asked one of the nurses to open the C-section kit and I squirted some betadine on the poor lady's abdomen. I gowned and gloved the best I could. Mostly for the baby, the mother was toast. I cut in the midline until I got down to the peritoneum. There wasn't much bleeding because the mother was about out of blood. Her pressure was so low that what little blood she had was hardly circulating. I entered the abdomen and easily located the very large uterus.

"Be careful Dr. Zander, the baby will be very close to the inner wall of the uterus. Open the uterus very cautiously or you will cut the baby," recommended the OB nurse.

That was welcome advice; I had never done one of these before.

I made a very small incision in the uterus and was met with a flood of amniotic fluid. The fluid was dark and contained yellow and brown material. I would later come to know that this was meconium from the baby being in distress. If I managed to birth this little sucker, we would have to get that shit out if its airway, or the meconium would mess up the lungs.

I poked a finger in the uterus and used that as a buffer between me and the baby. I then used blunt scissors to cut open the uterus. I pulled out the baby, who was blue and flaccid, and handed him to the nurse. The mother flatlined on the monitor and I elected not to pursue further resuscitation efforts with her. There was nothing to save except her legacy in the form of her baby. It was a girl.

The OB nurse frantically dried and stimulated the baby. She used a suction device to remove as much meconium from the child as she could.

"Do you want me to intubate her?" I asked.

"Dr. Zander please use a laryngoscope to help suction meconium from the airway. Do not intubate yet, or we will blow the meconium further in and damage the lungs."

I did as she said and suctioned the best that I could.

"Can you be a little gentler with the suction? We want to get as much meconium out without further irritating the airway," she said without any condescension.

"Will do." I knew she was right. It was hard to be gentle with all the adrenaline my body could produce coursing through my veins.

Once we got out as much as we could, I put a tube in the trachea so we could ventilate the patient. The child's oxygen saturation should have been close to 100% with the amount of oxygen we were delivering. But it was barely ninety percent. We needed some IV access to give some meds and antibiotics.

I had clamped and cut the umbilical cord for the delivery. Luckily, I had left about eight inches of it attached to the baby. The nurse suggested we insert an umbilical venous catheter. I trimmed about four inches off the umbilical cord and applied pressure to the cord to prevent any bleeding. The normal anatomy was two arteries and a vein. The vein was the smallest diameter of the three and we easily identified it. I held the cord as the nurse slipped in the catheter. We were in business.

After a couple rounds of resuscitation drugs, we infused double antibiotic coverage because of the unsterile conditions our baby experienced as she entered this world. To this pharmaceutical cocktail, we added two different drips of drugs to keep her blood pressure where we wanted. Crystal had prepared the drips in a miraculous timeframe. At this point, our baby was less blue and somewhat stable.

By this time, a number of surgeons and ER doctors had arrived because of the code violet. Buster, of all people, checked them in and allowed most of them to return home. Two of the ER doctors volunteered to stay. In the time that the resuscitations took, about ten new patients had arrived. One of the ER docs started to take care of them. The second ER doctor had been a pediatrician by training before her career in the ER. She volunteered to stay with the baby until the transport team from the Level Four NICU arrived. I kissed the OB nurse and Crystal on the cheek and headed to check on Hofucker.

CHAPTER 20

Emergency Department
Supreme Medical Center
0233 July 13

Deuce sat at the bedside holding Hofucker's hand, all the while crying like a baby. Dr. Stanton completed a phone call with the trauma center and walked over toward me.

He spoke, "The news is not good, but he is still alive and will likely survive."

His blood pressure was 100 and his oxygen saturation was ninety-two percent. Pretty good for most people. But he was getting a shitload of oxygen, and it should have been 100%. The CT scan of his head showed no evidence of clots, but there were multiple frontal areas injured. Unfortunately, those were suspicious for shear type injuries. They had the worst prognosis. With some mild hyperventilation, Hofucker was stable, but he needed an intracranial bolt and the care of skilled neurosurgeons. Fortunately, the trauma center reported that the weather in their direction was clearing. They had dispatched their chopper. The ETA was twenty minutes.

Dr. Stanton updated Deuce as I listened in. Hofucker had a severe right lung contusion in addition to multiple contusions and small lacerations of the liver. He had a large hematoma (blood clot) of his right kidney and a duodenal hematoma. He had fractures of his right arm and leg and multiple facial fractures.

This dude was in trouble. The big question was whether his brain injuries would allow him to survive? If he did, what would he be able to do? He might be lucky to talk without drooling, let alone ever practice medicine again. Then there was the matter of his being dickless. Sorry, but as a guy, you worry about shit like that.

The state police had arrived. To this point, they had been kept out of the room. Their biggest question was whether a blood alcohol level had been done. Jenny assured them that it had. It was their working theory that the driver of the truck had lost control of his vehicle and had caused the accident. But their investigation was at its infancy. One of the trooper's radios buzzed. The trooper left the room and returned looking even more shaken up than he had been before. His complexion was somewhere between pale and green.

"What is the identity of the patient in room four?" he inquired.

Jenny gave him Hofucker's driver's license that she had retrieved from his wallet. That matched the identity of the truck registration. The trooper copied down the information and looked up with a pained expression on his face.

"Did he have an injury to his penis?" he asked bashfully.

I replied, "As a matter of fact, it was amputated."

He stuttered slightly and said, "One of the troopers may have found it. A medic is transporting it to the ER. His ETA is 15 minutes."

I blurted out, "Thank goodness" before I knew what I had said.

Jenny gave me a stare that summed it up best. It said, "Great, the guy is half dead with serious brain injuries, and you are happy they found his dick! Men!"

We all stood in silence for a minute or so. I tried to figure out how Hofucker's member ended up in the street.

Just then, the trooper cleared his throat and said, "Do you have an employee named Marilyn?"

"Yes," shrieked Jenny.

The trooper asked us to sit down, and we quickly complied. He was slow and compassionate in his speech.

"I know you are both used to trauma and death but trust me you are never ready when it comes knocking on your door. We found a female victim of the accident along the side of the road. It appears that the truck rolled numerous times after impact. She was ejected from the vehicle and was dead. She was so badly injured that identification will be difficult. But we did find a purse nearby. In that purse we found an ID badge from Supreme Medical ER with the name of Marilyn Kucher. Would she have had any reason to be in Dr. Hofecker's truck?"

Jenny sobbed and could not speak. I hugged her tightly. After a few seconds, I told the officer that Marilyn was employed here and had a relationship with Dr. Hofecker. I think I had figured out why Hofucker lost control of his vehicle and how his manhood ended up on the pavers. But I wasn't making that speculation for the police. This thing was crazy enough.

CHAPTER 21

Emergency Department
Supreme Medical Center
0645 July 13

Hofucker arrived at the trauma center and our baby was admitted to the Level Four NICU. The stroke victim had regained full ability to talk and use his extremities.

"I owe you a beer," I said to Dr. Chew. Then I added, "I think I know your family."

"Really, who do you know?"

"Your sister Ah Chew, and your brother Fu Man Chew."

"You are half right; I am Fu Man. Fu Man Chew. That's what I was known by in college," he laughed.

Amos smiled as another nickname was born. Dr. Chew would be forever known as Fu Man in the ER, but he earned that moniker as a friend. He was a good dude, and he understood ER humor.

Amos and I walked slowly down the hall.

"Amos, was Hofucker drunk?" I asked, careful to keep my voice at a whisper.

"No question," he said. "I'd bet his blood alcohol concentration was 0.250 or higher."

0.080 was the legal limit. Amos was very good at the GTBAC game we also played in the ER: Guess The Blood Alcohol Content. Amos won quite often. Just then, Jenny walked toward us with Hofucker's labs hot off the printer.

"Jenny, did you get Hofucker's blood alcohol?"

"Yep, it was 47!"

"0.047???? Get the fuck out!" I said in shock.

Amos kicked me. I took that as a clue to hush.

Jenny just shook her head and continued her journey to the fax machine to send the results to the trauma center.

"Why did you kick me?" I asked Amos as we entered the employee lounge, which was empty.

"Doc ZZ, you are a cool dude, and I think you are an amazing doc. I also suspect that you and Jenny are a little closer than just coworkers. If you know what I mean."

I was about to profess my innocence when Amos continued.

"This isn't the first time in this ER that very drunk patients ended up with blood alcohol levels that were magically under the legal limit."

"What are you saying Amos? Who changed the lab result?" I inquired.

"Doc ZZ, I ain't saying nothin'. You're a smart dude. Figure it out."

Just then, Jenny opened the door to the lounge. "C'mon ZZ, we have to go to the morgue."

Jenny and I had to do the official identification. That could have been the most unpleasant thing I had ever done. On the way back from the morgue, we learned that the driver of the Prius was the husband of the mother. He was a decorated Marine who had only returned home from deployment a year ago. They had another daughter who was two. She was at her grandparents', and therefore avoided the accident. She and her newborn sister were now orphans. Life can really suck.

I was so tired that I had called Stephanie to get someone else to help with the horses. It was Sunday so they only needed to be fed, but I was in no shape to do anything. At least I was off today and there was no racing tonight. Jenny and I walked to our trucks together. We were both quiet, trying to process the events of the night.

"Thanks for all of your help tonight, you were just amazing," I added.

"Thanks, but I wish things had turned out better." She looked away because she was crying and didn't want me to see. Typical hard-ass ER nurse. I wanted to hold her and hug her, but I didn't.

"We got a good baby, Hofucker is likely to survive, and the dude with the stroke totally recovered. Sometimes, you have to see the good side."

I kissed her softly on top of her head. We went to our vehicles, drove to our respective homes, and collapsed into our beds.

CHAPTER 22

Barn 7

Miracle Mile Racetrack and Casino

0530 July 14

Sunday was a blur. I slept most of the day. Monday morning, I awoke at five and was at the track barn by 5:30. I saw Stephanie's truck and parked beside it. The engine was cold. She had been here for a while. I swear she worked twenty hours a day. As I entered, I noted that half of our barn had been watered and Stephanie was busy cleaning out her second stall. I stared at her while she worked, so petite and so cute. Five feet four inches of pure energy complimented by flowing blonde hair that hung clear down to her butt when she let it down. Today, it was stuffed under a Philadelphia Phillies baseball cap. Her jeans were muddy, and I am sure she smelled like a stable, but she was the sweetest thing.

I snuck up on her and pinched her ass.

She let out a scream and said, "Fuck you ZZ!"

She chased me down barn row with a pitchfork, laughing the whole time. Our game was interrupted by a crying infant who was carried into the barn by her mother. I didn't know her name, but I knew that her husband worked for Supreme Stables. I was pretty sure they were both illegal. In broken English, she explained that she had no money, and her baby was sick. Could I look at her? I knew the word had gotten out on the backstretch that I was back in town. In my younger days I was known to provide free medical care to anyone who couldn't afford a physician, which was half of the occupants of the backstretch.

I went to my truck and retrieved my little black bag. Yeah, I am one of the few docs that still had one. Stephanie cleaned off a table in the tack room and wiped it down with disinfectant. The baby had a fever of 102 but otherwise looked healthy. Her lungs were clear. Her throat looked good as did her right ear. The left eardrum was red, bulging, and about ready to burst. We had the culprit, but did we have the cure? People that can't afford a doctor usually can't afford medicine.

Unfortunately, I hadn't thought to purchase any antibiotics. I will take care of that omission today. I did manage to find some liquid Ibuprofen in the truck. I labeled and marked a syringe for the correct dose for a fever. I showed the mother how to administer it. I handed her a prescription for an antibiotic that I knew wasn't expensive. I also handed her a $10 bill to cover the cost. The mother cried and the baby stopped crying. Big win. In Spanish, I told her to call me if the baby got worse, and to have her grow up to be a doctor. She hugged me and left. Stephanie hugged me and then pricked my butt with the pitchfork.

We got done early and headed back to the farm. Stephanie wanted me to see the technique that she used to train our most difficult horses. She had been working with Fired Up Alabama for the past three months. She was a trotter who hadn't made it to the races at ages two and three. At two, she got sick and nearly died. At three, she had little nagging injuries that made her foul-gated and foul-spirited. She was a handful.

As Stephanie entered her stall, Alabama turned so her head faced the back corner of the stall. Then, she let both her back legs fly time and again.

"You want me, come get me," she was saying in horse speak.

I really hated it when horses did that. One wrong step and I could get another hoofprint scar on my face. Steph was unfazed. She juked to the right to miss the most recent volley of kicks and grabbed Alabama's halter. The horse tried to rear. Stephanie held her tight and rapped her on the head with her knuckle. Not too hard, but not too soft either. Big brown eyes met petite blue eyes, and all was calm. Stephanie turned her around then put her in crossties so she could get her equipment on.

"Her gait is much better. I found a way to calm her ass down on the track. I trained her down to 2:05. If she can do that today, I think she is ready to qualify."

I could not process what she had said. I was so amazed that she spoke so clearly, and without any F-bombs. I know her therapist had been working hard on her speech. Today is the first time I heard her complete a sentence that could be uttered on TV or the radio.

"Are you fucking listening to me?"

Ooopps, Stephanie did not appreciate my taking a few moments to analyze her speech. Old habits die hard, I thought.

"Of course, Stephanie, what did you do to get her to settle? I thought she would never make it to the races."

"Just watch."

She had Alabama ready in no time. She grabbed her helmet as she led Alabama out of the stall. She handed me a headset with a microphone. She got Alabama onto the track and jogged her a few miles to warm up. She turned her in the correct direction to train and I started to hear music.

The music was soft at first but grew louder as Stephanie approached the start line. Through the headset, I could hear Stephanie chirping to Alabama to get her up to speed. They passed the start line, and the music got louder. It was, of all things, "Sweet Home Alabama." For the first time I now noticed there were speakers about every fifty yards around the track.

I heard Stephanie singing as they trotted the first quarter in thirty seconds, which was what she wanted. I thought I remembered the words to the song, and I didn't remember them being the words I was hearing in my headset. "Sweet fucking home Alabama," Stephanie at her best.

I saw that a crowd had formed on the outside rail past the ¾ pole. They must have come from the Always Hope School. There were about 10 kids and 10 teachers and therapists.

"Stephanie, you have the army out early."

"That's my army. The Autistic Army. They have been helping me with Alabama."

"How's she feel, Steph?" I inquired.

"Pretty smooth," she said. Although it was hard to hear over the music, which by now was quite loud.

"Half in 102," Stephanie announced.

Since there were no F-bombs attached, I assumed she was happy with that.

As they hit the ¾ pole, I heard, "Get your lazy ass moving. Thirty-two, you should be ashamed."

I took that as displeasure at a third quarter that was slower than what Stephanie wanted. She popped the earplugs out, and Alabama took off.

Stephanie screamed, "Here comes the Army baby!!"

She rounded the turn at the top of the stretch, and I saw what she meant. All twenty kids and teachers were dancing to the music and putting their fists in the air and pulling them down. You know how kids ask truck drivers to blow their horns?

I saw Alabama glance to the outside. Stephanie put her arm in the air and pulled down as if she was blowing an 18-wheeler's horn. The kids kept dancing and gesturing and screaming. Stephanie let out a whoop. Alabama cut loose, trotting the last ¼ in twenty-seven seconds.

"Stephanie, you are amazing," I screamed into the mic.

"No, she is," (the horse), "and they are," (referring to the kids), "I'm just the dumb driver."

The music stopped. Stephanie jogged Alabama slowly around the track and stopped her at the rail near The Army. They screamed, they hollered, and they cried. Most of them couldn't talk but they didn't need to. It was easy to figure out what was on their minds. They loved this horse, and she loved them. Leave it to Stephanie to figure out how to tame a wild beast.

Speaking of Stephanie, she was one tough person to figure out. Some days she was downright yappy, albeit with a plethora of fucks and shits thrown into her word salad. Other days, she was locked in her room, so to speak. She didn't talk or even interact much. She grunted and avoided eye contact. I never knew what to expect when I saw her. As an ER doc, I had very little training about autistic kids. Some days, I wished I knew more so I could help her more. I had to sit down with the therapists and get more up to speed.

I walked with her as she cooled Alabama out and rubbed her down. Kids from the school were all through the barn with their teachers and therapist-handlers in tow. They really didn't accomplish much work, but they got a lot of therapy in. They got to groom some of the tamer horses. We had to groom them when they got done because they rarely finished a whole job, but they were making progress. It was amazing to see how many of them were smiling when they were in the barn. What a great sight.

"Will you qualify her for me ZZ?" Stephanie inquired as she finished up in Alabama's stall.

"Nope."

"Bullshit, why not?"

"Do it yourself," I replied.

"Huh?" Stephanie looked totally confused.

"I thought you and her should both qualify."

Earlier this year Stephanie had obtained her provisional driver's license. Then my dad got a shirt with a number on it, and things have been crazy since then. She hadn't driven in a race since he went to prison. We certainly had plenty to do now but I knew that Stephanie had talent. She knew horses and she was fearless. It was time for her to get her A-license. To get it, she had to drive in a number of parimutuel races to prove to the judges that she was competent and safe.

Alabama had never raced. She needed to qualify to show the judges that she had proper manners and enough talent to be competitive. Stephanie needed more drives, and a qualifier for Alabama would be a good start.

"ZZ, I don't think I'm totally ready," Stephanie said as she filled the water trough.

"I know you are Steph. Just drive her like you did today and you will be fine. You aren't scared, are you? "

"Nah, not really, I just don't want to embarrass you," she sighed.

"Stephanie, you never embarrass me. OK, sometimes you say things that I wish you hadn't, but I know you are working on that. I am incredibly proud of everything you do. Your life didn't start so well but you never complained. You have been a dream child for our parents, and I am proud to be your brother. Your guts and determination are an inspiration to me. I have never seen anyone work harder. I can't wait to see you perform on the track."

"Drop us in the box for next week," she screamed as she started stacking bales of hay.

I headed to the school for a sick call. Only one case today. Bite on the finger from another child. Not too bad but it had broken the skin. I'm sure there was a good story to go along with it, but the little guy wasn't talking today. I cleaned it up and gave his caretaker a prescription for an antibiotic.

"Bring him by tomorrow for a recheck," I added as I headed to the house.

CHAPTER 23

Fired Up Farms
1200 July 14

I had planned to take a nap to get ready for the races and a long night in the ER. Mom met me at the door as I walked into the house. I had forgotten my cell phone, and it was ringing all morning. Eventually, she answered it and wished she hadn't. She told me that the medical staff secretary demanded that I report to the hospital at 1 PM for an emergency meeting. My guess was that they were going to hang Buster out to dry. Good for the old prick, he deserved it. I looked at the time on my phone. It was noon. I showered, shampooed, and shaved, and made it there by 12:55 PM.

On the way to the hospital, I called Not Too Juicy Lucy. That was my nickname for the medical staff secretary. She was totally useless. She appeared much older than her stated age and looked like a dried-out prune. She had earned her nickname when Deuce first threatened me about my privileges. Not Too Juicy Lucy called me the next day and proceeded to tell me I needed to mind my Ps and Qs. I told her to eat shit. She seemed taken aback by that. Now, her assistant, also named Lucy, was a different matter. She was sweet and, if I do say so, gorgeous. She was nicknamed Juicy Lucy.

Not Too Juicy Lucy wouldn't tell me squat except that I needed to be in the medical staff conference room at 1 PM. She never did like me. I always suspected that Mr. Penie or maybe Mrs. Penie hadn't visited her in a while. I didn't know for sure, but I probably was right. Some women get downright mean when it's been too long. And this bitch was nasty.

At 1 PM, I walked into the conference room and there sat the executive committee of the medical staff. That was composed of the heads of every clinical department. All departments were represented except emergency medicine. Janet wasn't there. I was directed to a seat near the front of the table. The meeting was being conducted by Buster. You know, Dr. Hyman. He looked tired and pissed off.

As soon as my ass hit the seat, Buster started to bellow in the monotone that he was famous for. He looked exceptionally old today, much older than his sixty years. His eyes were baggy and bloodshot, and he had a tremor of the hand he was holding some papers in. Clearly, he was running this witch hunt, and I appeared to be the object of his ire.

"Dr. Zander, you are hereby notified of a summary suspension of your privileges, pending a full investigation by a subgroup of this committee. Until this matter is properly adjudicated, you are banned from the practice of medicine in this facility. You are further barred from entering the facility, except for attending proceedings relative to this matter."

"And what matter is that, Buster?" I shouted.

"Don't call me Buster, you heathen. If you can keep your mouth shut for a few minutes, I will be happy to read to you the charges," mumbled Buster with a wry smile on his face. He then continued. "You are not permitted to enter the facility except as a patient, or as needed to present a defense to your case. You are not permitted to discuss the case with anyone who was not involved in it. You are not permitted to discuss the case with anyone who was involved in it unless a member of the investigative committee is present. Although you will have the ability to request copies of meeting minutes and other documents for your defense, I will have the final say as to which documents are appropriate for you to access. Please refer to the medical staff bylaws Section A.4 for the rules of summary suspension. Do you have any questions?"

I really wanted to ask how many times he got butt humped in grade school, but I decided to hold that one for later. I raised my voice and said, "What are the charges?"

Buster recited them as if he said them every day, "1. Wrongful death of patient Cynthia Walker. You might know her as Jane Doe, the pregnant woman from the accident. Not only did you not listen to my advice, but you countermanded my order to the medics to take her to the trauma center. You diverted her here so you could do a C-section to look like a hero to your staff and medics. Had she been taken directly to the trauma center; she might have survived. It was highly likely that her baby would have been born under more appropriate conditions."

My face was purple. I stood and screamed; "Bullshit" as loud as I could.

Just then a Grange County deputy sheriff jumped up from his seat and yelled at me, "Calm down, shut up, and get back in your seat."

He had his hand on his taser. I know that Buster was hoping he would get the chance to use it. I sat back down. Buster smiled and continued.

"2. Inappropriate emergency C-section. You lacked the training and privileges necessary for the procedure. You should have stabilized the mother and transferred her immediately to a tertiary obstetrics center. 3. Loss of potential donated organs. Cynthia was an organ donor. You should have stabilized her as best as possible to preserve her organs for transplant. 4. Wrongful death of Marilyn Kucher."

I couldn't help myself and screamed, "How the hell is that possible? She was dead on arrival!"

Deputy Taser was at my side again, but he seemed happy with the fact that I didn't leave my seat.

Buster droned on, "You witnessed an inappropriate interaction between the deceased and Dr. Hofecker. You admonished Dr. Hofecker, but never reported the incident of moral turpitude as was required by the rules and regulations. Had you done so, the deceased likely would have refrained from performing a sex act on Dr. Hofecker as he drove the night of the accident. His blood alcohol concentration was only 0.047. The police conclusion is that he lost control of the vehicle when he climaxed. The accident was totally preventable."

"You have to be shitting me. Is this some kind of dream? An alternative universe? Do the rest of you concur with this crap?" I asked the other members of the committee.

No response. They sat there like the zombies they were.

Buster resumed reading from the papers now shaking badly in his severely trembling hands. I'd hate to see that dude's bar bills. And this guy operates on people?

"5. Inflicting emotional distress on Dr. Hofecker and Marilyn Kucher causing them to consume alcohol on the night of the accident. He fortunately had only a minimal amount, but she consumed far too much. Dr. Hofecker stated that she had been drinking heavily since the night of the incident in the ER. Her inebriation undoubtably contributed to her decision to provide oral sexual gratification to Dr. Hofecker as he operated a vehicle. 6. HIPPA violation. Divulging Dr. Hofecker's pelvic trauma to the police without a warrant. Add to the list charge 7. Inappropriate conduct at this meeting including disrespect for medical staff officers, rude and foul language, threatening speech, and behaviors."

I shrieked, "This is preposterous! Why not blame me for the spread of cancer or the heartbreak of psoriasis. I did more to cause those things than any of this bullshit."

Buster responded. "You will have your opportunity to answer these charges in due time. Going forward, you must conduct yourself in a proper manner. Please note that you will be removed from any meeting in which you cause a disturbance. Finally, you are officially informed that if you are found guilty of any of these charges your case will be referred to the state medical board. You could have your medical license revoked or sanctioned."

"Does anyone else here smell how bad this is?" I asked.

No one answered. They just stared at their navels and kept silent.

"May I go now, Buster?"

He nodded. I guessed he was getting used to his nickname. I stood and walked to the door with Deputy Taser on my heels. He followed me the whole way to my truck. I got in the truck and ground down the window.

"Let me tell you something deputy, if you step over the line of the law once with me, I will have your badge."

He laughed. "Pretty tough words from the son of a drunk murderer." He turned and walked back into the hospital.

128

CHAPTER 24

On the way home, I tried to reach Jenny to cancel our date. She never answered her phone. Maybe they had gotten to her, and she wasn't talking to me. Since I wasn't allowed back in the hospital, she might have to do a few errands for me.

The traffic was terrible due to some construction. That gave me plenty of time to ponder the charges and how bogus they were. Cynthia would never have survived to make it to the trauma center, nor would her baby. I should be congratulated for saving the baby. But now I am being made out as an egotistical asshole who did a bunch of stuff to look cool.

The worst was the bullshit with Hofucker. No, I didn't report the coitus in the gyne room. But what if I had? Would Dr. Hyman have lectured him and Marilyn on the time and place for sex? Would he have covered the dangers of driving while having an orgasm? Hardly. The only things on that list that I was guilty of were the conduct issues. Buster was lucky he had Deputy Taser standing by or he might have been busted up.

What a mess. We were six weeks from the Miracle Mile Millions, and I had almost zilch in race money. Without the ER job, I would have no other income. I had four weeks to come up with six million, or we lost the farm and Always Hope. And, I had to defend myself against these charges and hope not to lose my medical license.

I got home and told Mom and Stephanie. Mom sobbed and Stephanie balled up her fists and chanted "motherf'ers" repeatedly.

"What are you going to do Zachary?" Mom asked. She's the only person on the earth that called me Zachary.

Unlike most times, I did not have an answer, either correct or smartass. I went to my room. There was only one instance in my life when things were this hopeless, and therein lied the answer. There are times that you need the help of others. I got on my computer and searched for my list of contacts. I copied down the numbers for three. I called them, one at a time, and got voice mail each time.

I left the same message for all three. "Dying Was Easy, Fired Up Farm 1774 Marigold Lane, Krenshaw NJ 02006. Call me if you have any questions. If not, rendezvous at 1500 this Thursday July 17 at the above address."

I wondered if any or all of them would come. Time would tell.

I walked down to the kitchen and kissed Mom. She was still sobbing. Stephanie was waiting for me. She wanted me to walk with her. Since she had stopped chanting, we walked silently to the barn and right to Always Hope's stall Stephanie stroked her mane and looked at me.

"ZZ," she said.

"Guilty," I replied.

"No ZZ, no funnies, no jokes. I want you to know that this is where I come when I am as low as I can go. Those are the times when I look at other people and know that I'm a retard."

"Steph, don't you EVER say that again."

"Say what you want ZZ, but I know I am not normal. I don't think right, I don't talk right. I dream about being like other kids. And when I get really fucking low, I come here. This big mare talks to me. She says that being tough starts with your heart, not your mind or your body. Then after that you have to work and work hard. You drove her, you know. Quit wasn't a word she knew. Call me an asshole but I try to be like her."

"You are like her. You are tough, and you are beautiful. You are different, but so was she. She was a freak of a horse but she used her difference to her advantage. Don't ever try to be someone else Steph. We all love you the way you are."

"ZZ, I know you did what was right that night in the ER. I also know that Mom and I will help you fight this. Just like Always Hope did, we will find a way to win."

Stephanie started crying again, but that was interrupted by my phone ringing.

It was Crystal. She had been fired.

"What the hell for?" I asked.

"When I came to the ER to help with your C-section and resuscitation, I left the pharmacy unattended. I took my pager, but with all the noise and confusion in the resuscitation room I didn't hear it. When I got back to the pharmacy, I realized that I had missed a page from ICU. One of the patients needed a versed drip. I called immediately when I got back to the pharmacy and rushed the med to ICU. The nurse wasn't upset at all, even though she waited over forty-five minutes to get the drug. Well today I got pulled into the committee reviewing your handling of the C-section. They were quite unhappy that I totally supported you. Of course, they implied that I, as a pharmacist, would have no knowledge of anything except the drugs involved. However, I told them that I knew a moribund patient when I saw one, and this patient was not salvageable. Her drugs to support her as an organ donor had been maxed out and in my opinion her organs would have never been able to be donated. That is when they brought up the versed drip. But this time they had a written statement from the same nurse indicating that the delay in receiving the medication almost cost the patient his life. I was terminated after that statement was read."

"You will of course challenge this!" I demanded.

"No, Dr. Zander, I won't." Crystal softly answered. "Although I dispute the fact that the patient nearly died, my failure did delay his receiving a needed medication."

I stuttered, "But c'mon, there were extenuating circumstances!"

"I know," she said. "But they got me dead to rights, particularly now with the nurse's revised statement. So, I am taking some time off."

"What are you going to do?"

"Well, I was thinking of having my stomach stapled, and then applying for a one-year program with ISMP (Institute for Safe Medical Practices.) I really want to help with research on preventable medical errors. I have been contemplating the surgery for a while. I was hoping for a drug to come along that would help me with my weight problem, but I think the surgery is my best long-term answer."

"I sure will miss you at the hospital. Well, if I ever get back in the hospital, I will miss you."

"Thank you, Dr. Zander. It has been my pleasure to work with you."

"Can you stop at the farm sometime before you leave? The staff want to thank you for managing the prophylaxis for the meningitis case. By the way, the child appears to be doing well. Children's expects a full recovery. They credit your help with the selection and dosing of the antibiotic as a major factor in his positive outcome."

"I wish I could, but I have a flight out to Minneapolis tomorrow. I will be having my surgery there and when I recover, I will head to ISMP headquarters. I will stay in touch. You haven't seen the last of me."

"I hope not. Good luck and God bless you."

"Good luck to you Dr. Zander. You are going to need it with those fools at Supreme Medical. Oh, I almost forgot the main reason I called."

"What was that?" I inquired.

"I am not sure what to make of it. When I was waiting to be interviewed by the committee, I was seated in the hall around the corner from the door to the conference room. All of sudden I heard the door open and there was some activity in the hall. I couldn't see the people involved, nor could they see me. However, I recognized the voices as those of Dr. Hyman and Mr. Hofecker. Mr. Hofecker was really ticked off. He was half screaming at Dr. Hyman."

I asked, "What was he saying?"

"Something to the effect of, 'You better bury that little shit, Zander. Get all of his licenses suspended as soon as possible. Make sure that they stay suspended until September 1.' Dr. Hyman questioned whether he could pull it off. Mr. Hofecker did not want to hear it. I can tell you exactly what Mr. Hofecker said this time because I wrote it down. He said, 'Look you old drunk. Get it done, and make it stick, or your days on the gravy train are over.'"

"Whoooah," I said.

"I thought it might help your cause to know. You take care of yourself. Goodbye for now."

CHAPTER 25

Medical Staff Office
Supreme Medical Center
1000 July 15

Those assholes were planning on having my hearing the next day. A lynching was more like it.

"Why so soon? And what the hell do you mean that I can't bring my attorney?" I screamed.

"ZZ, please keep your voice down. Not Too Juicy Lucy will have my head if she finds out you were alone in this office with me. You are not to have any contact with any hospital employees without a medical staff chaperone present."

"Juicy Lucy, I apologize for my language. I was just so upset." I couldn't help but notice Juicy Lucy's short short skirt had exposed most of her long wraparounds. Mr. G suggested further exploration of the subject matter. See what I mean about him? Never stops. A cooler head prevailed. I was in enough trouble.

"Dr Zander, you tear me up. No apology is necessary. Between you and I, I think you are being screwed big time. They know how to play the game. They don't want you to have time to prepare a defense. Not Too Juicy Lucy's dehydrated head is so far up Buster's ass that she can taste his aftershave. But I wanted to explain as much as I can about the process to help you. I know that she is meeting with the Executive Committee for the next hour and that she won't be back until at least 11 AM."

"I really appreciate your support. But seriously, I don't get an attorney?"

"Not for the hearing. You can for the appeal if you lose and want one. If you lose, you definitely want an appeal."

"Why is that?" I asked.

"You do know about NJ SB 12.74?"

"Lucy, I have a lot better things to do than to pay attention to the crap done by New Jersey legislators."

"You might want to bone up on this item. All physicians supposedly got an email. But if you didn't, the law and an explanation of how it affects NJ physicians is on the medical board website."

"Can you give me the Cliffs notes?"

"Sure. If any medical institution or insurer suspends your privileges, they are required to immediately notify the state board of medicine. They, in turn, will suspend your medical license for sixty days while they investigate the matter. The medical board can reinstate your license, revoke your license, or impose restrictions on your license. However, any suspension of your medical license causes an automatic, and immediate, suspension of all licenses issued by the state. That would include driver's licenses and any licenses you have pertaining to racing. Those also remain suspended for sixty days while those licensing boards or bodies review the reason for the medical license suspension. They are required to determine if that problem or behavior should result in a loss or reductions of privileges for other licenses."

"But didn't they already suspend me? Are my medical license and other licenses suspended."

"No, not yet. It's not that they didn't try. Not Too Juicy Lucy was on the phone with the State Board this morning. Your privileges to practice here are suspended but your licenses are still valid. They will not be suspended until the morning after your hearing, if they uphold the charges. Which they will."

"That is absurd!!!!"

"Do you remember the Dagostino case?"

"Wasn't that the physician's assistant that sexually assaulted a patient and then later sexually assaulted someone he massaged?"

"Yes, he had a physician's assistant license and a massage therapist license. There was a big kerfuffle after he was convicted of the massage assault. It occurred two months after the medical board suspended his license while investigating the medical sexual assault. The plaintiff in the massage assault, and the media, felt that the massage assault could have been prevented had the massage therapist license been suspended pending the investigation of the medical license."

"There is some logic to that, but it doesn't really apply to my case."

"True, but you know the legislature. Act first, and figure out the details later, especially in an election year."

"So, when they find me guilty on some or all of the charges, I am totally screwed."

"Only half screwed. Your medical license and all other licenses will be suspended on the next business day for sure. However, the suspension can be stayed if you file an appeal, and the appeal is completed within thirty days. During the time prior to completion of the appeal all licenses remain active."

"Then I am not screwed if I appeal?"

"You still are because Deuce and Buster, as you call them, will schedule the appeal for forty-five days or so from now to trigger the suspensions. To get the stay, you have to show that the appeal will be done in thirty days."

I decided to cross that bridge when it came and to concentrate on the hearing. If I won at the hearing, there would be no suspensions. Juicy Lucy explained that I was allowed to bring a support person to the hearing, but they had to be a member of the medical staff.

She concluded with, "Be in conference room two at 6 PM tomorrow. Let me know if I can help you in ANY way but keep it between us. Good luck."

I sensed that there was some hidden meaning to that statement. My level of suspicion increased when Juicy Lucy bent down to put her copy of the bylaws in the bottom drawer of the filing cabinet. I was pretty sure she had obtained it from the top drawer. Hats off to the inventor of thong underwear.

CHAPTER 26

Greengate Apartments
Daquiri Hill, NJ
1600 July 15

Luck might be the only thing that could save me. Another ER doctor, Gerry Martines, agreed to be my support person. He was two months from retirement and had nothing to lose. Plus, he hated Buster with a passion. Apparently, Buster screwed him on a case a few years back. He told me how the hearing was likely to go. He watched a few other doctors get thrown off staff. That was how it was done at Supreme. If you were not with the in-crowd or appeared to be against them, you were destined for the door.

Gerry was not surprised with how quickly the hearing was scheduled. "They do that, so you can't mount much of defense."

I was pissed. "That's damn unfair. How do they get away with that shit?"

"Pretty simple, they claim you are incompetent and likely to hurt more patients if you are permitted to keep practicing."

"What else can you tell me about this trial?" I needed to know all I could.

"If they have an open and shut case, they use a hearing panel. Which is a minimum of three docs, one of which must be from your specialty. If they don't have an airtight case, they use a 'hearing officer' instead of a hearing panel." Gerry paused for a minute for emphasis.

"What difference does that make?" I quipped.

"One whole hell of a lot. The hearing officer does not have to be a physician. In fact, it almost always is some attorney well paid by the hospital."

"So?"

"When it comes to clinical decisions, like emergency C-sections and whether a patient is an organ donor, wouldn't you rather be judged by peers versus a snake?"

"You call attorneys snakes too?" I laughed nervously.

"Hopefully, you will laugh when this is over. ZZ they are going to rake you over the coals and do their best to bust up your career. These people play for keeps."

"OK, spell it out for me."

"When they use a hearing officer, he or she runs the meeting like a judge. This is essentially a trial before a judge. They present their case by calling various members of the medical staff to present the charges. You get to cross-examine them if you wish."

"Do I get to call any defense witnesses?"

"Sure, you do. You can call any member of the medical staff. But just so you know, it's likely that no one will testify for you except me. The rest of the sheep are too far away from retirement to have any balls."

"Can I call Janet Dawson?" (The ED director)

"Sure, if she shows up. Oftentimes, key potential witnesses for the defense seem to be out of town or otherwise unable to testify."

"But your testimony will be key."

"Not necessarily. The hearing officer will likely say that I am biased. So, he cannot totally accept what I have to say. It's bullshit but they that is how they do it. You will be found guilty on most of the charges. They usually let you skate on one or two to make it look good. But the most serious ones will stick, and you will be thrown off staff."

"Can you be any more negative?"

"Just painting the picture, my friend. Your best chance of getting out of this happens in your appeal. That goes to the board of directors, and you get to have an attorney. But don't get your hopes up too much. They use a hearing panel, and one has to be a physician, but not necessarily an ER doc. But they also can use a hearing officer instead of the panel. It's a safe bet that they will go the hearing officer route for the appeal."

"What about fairness and due process?" I protested.

"I wouldn't expect either of those if I was you," Gerry replied.

CHAPTER 27

Executive Conference Room
Supreme Medical Center
1745 July 16

Gerry and I arrived at 5:45 PM. We sat in the hall and made small talk as we waited for our grand entrance. At exactly 6 PM, the door opened and there sat the entire executive committee of the medical staff, minus one. Conspicuously absent was Janet Dawson, the chairperson of the ER. I knew right away that the fix was in. If she was in the room, I could call her as a witness. They knew she would not be able to support the charges, so they got her to take a powder. I guess that bitch liked her job and perks more than she did her profession. A whore by any other name. The room was just packed with them.

Deputy Taser was there along with Buster and his friends. We were directed to a table which had been set before a large desk. They had tried to make the room look like a courtroom. At the "prosecution table" sat Buster and Roy Bator. Roy is a neurosurgeon. Talk about a strange group, neurosurgeons. Most of them were way too smart but also way too arrogant. Roy was top in his class in both categories. No wonder they always said in medical school that the neurosurgeons were the kids no one would play with in kindergarten. I affectionately had nicknamed Roy "Master." He was known in the ER as "Master Bator."

Buster rose and called meeting to order. The jagoff even had a large gavel. What a show. The remainder of the executive committee settled into seats in the gallery. Buster began in that monotone drawl for which he was famous.

"The purpose of the hearing is to adjudicate the summary suspension of Dr. Zachary Zander. Per section A of the medical staff bylaws I, with the concurrence of the CEO Mr. Hofecker, have appointed Eiton Shapiro ESQ as a hearing officer. He will conduct the hearing and deliver a verdict on each charge. Are there any objections?" He handed the gavel to Shapiro.

I slowly stood and did my best to stay composed. "I object on the basis that a layman is being asked to pass judgment on medical decisions. He has no training or further qualifications to rule on areas of medical judgment."

"Overruled!" erupted a deep voice that had been hidden in the massively obese body that belonged to Mr. Shapiro.

"Judges and juries daily make decisions on liability, medical errors, patent disputes, etcetera that they have no specific knowledge about. The court process allows them to be educated through the trial and then express their opinion as to the facts of the case. That is the foundation for the rule of law in this country."

I think he wanted to rant on further, but he appeared to have run out of breath. If he passed out, I wouldn't plan on helping him. Sorry Hippocrates. Maybe Buster could resuscitate him by waving a Twinkie under his nose.

I had a smile on my face as I asked, "And how many of those decisions were flat-out wrong?" The grin was unintentional, but I couldn't help it. Mr. Shapiro's nickname just erupted from my frontal cortex. Eat A Ton Shapiro, how appropriate and funny. Gallows humor, I guess. I didn't call him that, but I was surely thinking it. As a physician, I have compassion for severely overweight patients. Their lives are often short and mostly unpleasant. But I have no love lost for pricks trying to do me in. Eat A Ton was in the latter category. I wondered if he was a mind reader. He got a second wind and unloaded on me.

"Dr. Zander you are facing serious charges here. Just so we understand each other, I will not tolerate any outbursts or malicious behavior such as you exhibited before this distinguished group of colleagues in the past. Am I clear?"

"When I see a group of distinguished colleagues, I will behave myself. But for now, you are shit out of luck."

Out of the corner of my eye, I saw Deputy Taser lift his fat ass out of his comfortable chair. Gerry rolled his eyes and looked at the floor.

"One more interruption or vulgarity and I will have you removed," bellowed Eat A Ton.

"Well then, bring in the kangaroos, so we can get this kangaroo court in motion."

My ears were split by the sound of the large gavel pounding on the table.

"Order, order," screamed Eat A Ton. "We will take the charges one by one. I would like to start with the least serious charges and work our way up. Dr. Hyman, please read charge seven."

"Inappropriate conduct at an official medical staff meeting involving disrespect for medical staff officers, rude and foul language, threatening speech, and offensive behavior."

Eat A Ton peered over his glasses. "Dr. Zander, how do you plead?"

"I plead guilty to all except the threatening speech. I did indeed show disrespect for the medical staff officers, and I still have no respect for them. Pompous asses one and all, but I never threatened anyone."

Eat A Ton appeared pleased. "Would there be any objection from the medical staff if the phrase threatening speech was removed from the charges?"

Buster replied, "His demeanor was threatening to me, but in the spirit of a quick and fair proceeding, the medical staff agrees to drop the charge of threatening speech."

Gerry nodded his head as if to say, "See, I told you so."

Eat A Ton continued, "Very good, the defendant is found guilty of charge seven with the revised language. I trust Dr. Zander, that you will see that this process is fair and efficient. Let's proceed with charge six, inappropriate HIPPA violation. Dr. Zander did you disclose the nature of Dr. Hofecker's penile injury to the police?"

"I did sir."

"Guilty."

"I object. The disclosure was necessary for his ongoing care. That disclosure to the police allowed for his amputated penis to be transferred with him to the trauma center where it was subsequently reattached."

"Overruled. Guilty on charge six."

Eat A Ton obviously hadn't seen his own crank for quite a while so he must have thought this was no big deal. I wanted to argue this point further, but we had bigger fish to fry.

On charge four, wrongful death of Marilyn Kucher, I was pleased with a mixed verdict. Eat A Ton dismissed the wrongful death charge. Even he thought it was a stretch that by my not reporting them that I caused her death. He refused to accept the testimony of the chief of psychiatry, Dr. Stanley Hershberger. AKA in the ER as Hash. (He supposedly was a cannabis freak.) Hash stated that he was sure that he could have counseled Dr. Hofecker and Marilyn, and that the accident could have been avoided. Did I mention that Hash was Buster's brother-in-law? Funny coincidence.

But I didn't escape with a clean slate. He found me guilty of not reporting the sexual incident I witnessed as was required by the rules and regulations. I'll take that hit any day.

OK, guilty on three minor charges, and not guilty on one major. Three to go.

"Charge three. Loss of potential donated organs."

Buster rambled on. "Everyone knows that organ donation saves lives. Countless patients were robbed of a chance at continued life when Dr. Zander made his fatal decision. He sentenced them to die when he directed the ambulance come to Supreme ER instead of proceeding directly to the trauma center."

"I totally disagree with everything Buster just uttered. I strongly object to the inflammatory language he used. His conclusions are pure bullshit."

Eat A Ton admonished me, "Dr. Zander, there is no place for profanity or name-calling in this hearing. Dr. Hyman, please continue, but do tone down the rhetoric a little please."

That sickening monotone began again. "The trauma center was an organ donor center. They were equipped to harvest organs in a short period of time. The delay incurred when Ms. Walker was brought to Supreme ER resulted in her premature death, and loss of organs. At a minimum, she should have been maintained on life support until she could have been sent to the trauma center."

"Dr Zander?"

"I totally disagree. This patient was moribund. Her chance of survival was zero. She had been maxed out on all supportive drugs, and her blood pressure was incredibly low despite that. Her organs were not being perfused and were not going to be salvageable."

Buster interrupted. "There were surely other drugs that you should have used to raise her blood pressure, were there not? But you were so focused on botching an emergency C-section to impress your staff, and feed your ego, that you ignored them."

"Look you prick!"

Before I could finish the gavel rapped and Eat A Ton screamed, "Dr. Zander you are one step from being removed."

"Sorry Mr. Shapiro, but Dr. Hyman insisted on using provocative language such as botching a surgical procedure, and ignoring life-saving drugs, that I lost control." I was proud of myself for calling him Mr. Shapiro.

"Continue," he replied.

"Crystal Johns, our pharmacist, confirmed that we had maxed out the pressor agents, the drugs used to raise her blood pressure."

Buster objected. "The pharmacist in question is not here for us to cross-examine. In fact, she was fired for her actions on the night in question."

Eat A Ton rapped the gavel and said, "Let's deal with what testimony we can elicit from the people in this room. For this hearing, we can only rely on who is present. Dr. Zander, you may continue."

"Cynthia Walker possibly could have donated her organs if a helicopter had been able to take her from the scene directly to a trauma center. When that wasn't possible, I had the medics bring her to Supreme Medical to deliver her baby. Had we been able to stabilize her, I would have sent her on to the trauma center for organ donation. Unfortunately, she did not make it."

Buster responded, "Your decision to bring her here was based upon your ego, and desire to be seen as a hero by your staff."

"Bull–!" I pulled the shit from the phrase just in time. "Mr. Shapiro, the loss of the patient's organs was the result of her injuries coupled with poor weather conditions precluding prompt evacuation to the trauma center."

Shapiro seemed to listen.

"I will rule on this charge after I hear testimony on charge one. Let's examine charge one now. The wrongful death of Cynthia Walker, Dr. Bator?"

Master stood. After an uncomfortable pause, he pulled out the cheapest-looking reading glasses I ever saw. Warby Parker's they were not. They were the kind that broke down in the middle, and he played with them for a long time. Then he began. He had a shrill voice that was as welcoming as fingernails on a chalkboard. He rambled on and on in complex neurosurgical and anatomical terms to impress all involved. All I could think was that he was a flaming arrogant asshole. If you look that up, I guarantee you will find his picture. After a protracted and incredibly boring presentation, he concluded.

"Cynthia Walker was salvageable. But any chance she had at life went down the drain when she was not taken by ambulance directly to the trauma center. The intervention a properly trained neurosurgeon may have made an incredible difference."

Eat A Ton looked in my direction, "Dr. Zander?"

"Dr. Bator," I really wanted to call him Master. But I was about to castrate him, and I didn't want to miss my chance by getting the boot. "Are you a properly trained neurosurgeon?"

Master rose and grinned, "You know my credentials are impeccable."

Time to explode the grenade. "Then why did you not save Cynthia? You did come to the hospital that night, did you not?"

Buster nervously jumped to his feet. "He arrived after you gave up on the patient. There was no need for him to evaluate her."

Only two people knew that Master was checked in and excused at 1:05 AM. I was one and Juicy Lucy was the other. She observed Not Too Juicy Lucy making a copy of something that looked like a sign-in sheet for the Code Violet. It had a purple band at the top. She then saw her throw the original in the confidential trash bin to be shredded. Juicy Lucy turned the bin upside down and retrieved the document after Not Too Juicy went home.

I pulled the document from my pocket and read, "Dr. Bator was checked in for the Code Violet at 1:05 AM. I pronounced Cynthia Walker at 2:05 AM. If anyone could have saved her, Dr. Bator, a self-proclaimed world-class neurosurgeon, could have done it. Except he went home before she even arrived."

That brought the house down. Eat A Ton called for a recess to try to sort things out. I quickly adjourned to the bathroom to relieve a badly engorged bladder. A short time later I was joined by Gerry.

He laughed as he said, "You got them on the run. I had no idea that Dr. Bator had been there that night. You sure made him look like the creep that he is."

Our discussion was interrupted by Deputy Taser, who grunted and pointed for us to return to the conference room. Eat A Ton looked uber pissed. I was hoping that he was just jonesing for a Snickers. No such luck.

He cut loose, "Dr. Zander you appear intent upon making a mockery of these proceedings. I will have no more of it. For your information, the sign-in sheet that you illegally obtained had been discarded because it was inaccurate. Dr. Bator did not respond to the ER until 3:02 AM. Dr. Hyman made an error when he recorded the time.. The medical staff secretary discovered the mistake the next day and revised the sheet for accuracy. You owe Dr. Bator and this body an apology."

Amos swore to me that he saw Dr. Bator's car leaving the doctor's parking lot at 1:30 AM. When Amos's friend in security tried to access the log of keycard entries and exits from the doctor's lot for that night, he found that it had been deleted. I could find no one else that saw the exact time the little worm arrived that night. I knew Buster was lying but I was screwed.

"I refuse to apologize but I am willing to move on."

Eat A Ton accepted my terms.

"Dr. Zander do you wish to call any witnesses at this time?"

"Yes, I would like to call Janet Dawson, my supervisor and ER director."

"Is she present in this room?"

"No, I have been trying to reach her and I have not been able to locate her. Her secretary does not know where she is. She was to work in the ER tonight but got someone to cover for her."

"Well, you can't have someone testify who is not here, can you? Anyone else?"

"I would like to have Gerry Martines testify."

"I object," shouted Buster as he leaped out of his seat. "Gerry Martines is a loyal friend of Dr. Zander. He is hardly an objective witness. Dr. Martines is biased against me. I brought charges against him years ago over an ectopic pregnancy that he missed in the ER."

"Sustained," Shapiro hammered the gavel. "I cannot believe this witness will be credible due to his bias. He will not testify."

Gerry and I went ballistic. The room erupted with profanity-laden insults and threats. This time, it took fifteen minutes and a backup car of sheriff's deputies to restore order.

Shapiro rapped the gavel. "I have instructed the deputies to detain anyone making any further statements or interrupting me, and I mean it. So, everyone sit down, and shut up. I am shocked at the things I heard tonight and the behavior of what are supposed to be learned professionals. I will tolerate it no more. I am prepared to rule on all counts."

I stood and calmly said, "But we haven't concluded testimony, and we have…."

Shapiro screamed, "Deputies place Dr. Zander in custody."

Two deputies with bad haircuts grabbed me and threw me to the ground. After handcuffing me, they stood me up. One of them noticed Dr. Martines filming the encounter, and they seized his phone. He then was also handcuffed.

Shapiro smirked as he said, "If either of you two wants to be gagged, just speak up now."

There was silence.

"Good choice. As I said, I am prepared to announce my rulings. Considering the written proffers and live testimony of your peers, I conclude that your judgments and actions in managing the cases described did not meet the high standards required by the bylaws of Supreme Medical. Your behavior, and that of your support person, further underscores the fact that you are unfit to practice in a highly functional and respected institution such as this. I find you responsible for the death of Cynthia Walker. I find that you performed an emergency C-section that you were not properly trained or credentialed for. Your actions and decisions that night caused a loss of donated organs. You committed a HIPPA violation by disclosing protected health information. You failed to report an incident of moral turpitude as was required by the rules and regulations. I affirm the medical staff's request for your privileges to be revoked, and hereby remove you from the medical staff. This action will be reported to the State Board of Medicine tomorrow at 9 AM in compliance with NJ SB 12.74. And Dr. Martines, you will face charges due to your behavior tonight. I would ask for your responses, but I don't care to hear them. Deputies, take them away."

CHAPTER 28

Holding Cell
Krenshaw Police Department
2030 July 16

"I told you this would not turn out well," Gerry said as we sat in the corner of the cell.

"You were right," I said. "Sorry to have gotten you involved."

"Well, it is something to tell the grandkids about. I am starting my retirement tomorrow. No sense fighting these assholes. What are you going to do?"

"First, I am going to get my ass out of here. I hope they get here for bail soon. I recognize a couple of guys on the other side of the room. I am pretty sure that they were previous winners in the asshole of the night contest."

Without staring, Martines says, "Yep, you are right. One of them looks like Jimmy Fulton, the current undisputed title holder for the award. Turn away from them so we don't make eye contact."

A few minutes later, an officer came to the cell and motioned for us to exit. We gladly complied. After signing a bunch of papers, we were met by Mom in the lobby.

I began an explanation of the night's proceedings as we walked to the car. We dropped Gerry at his house, and on the way home, I explained the rest of the bad news to Mom. Not only was I suspended from practicing medicine but my license to own, train and drive horses was suspended.

Mom sobbed, "That doesn't make sense."

By the time I explained the Dagostino case and the resulting laws that had been passed we arrived home. Mom had told Stephanie that I had been arrested. Apparently, Stephanie went bonkers. Mom was worried she would cause a scene at the police station, so she had one of the therapists from the school sit with her while Mom sprung us.

I walked to Stephanie's room to say good night. I thanked the therapist and allowed her to return to the school. Stephanie was sitting in her rocking chair facing the corner. She was chanting choice expletives. My eyes filled with tears. I wiped them dry as I closed her door behind me. There was no use trying to communicate with her until she stopped chanting. Previous efforts to do so had gotten me injured. I had enough for today.

But there was no limit on the pain that I would inflict on those who messed with my family. Stephanie had made significant gains with her speech. Someone is going to pay a hefty price for sending her back to chanting.

CHAPTER 29

Fired Up Farms
1335 July 17

Mom told me that Stephanie stopped chanting at 3 AM. She was still at the track by 0530. I got four more hours of sleep, but my ass was still dragging. Somehow, we got our work at the barn done and were home by noon.

Stephanie had fallen fast asleep on the couch. She was abruptly awakened by a knock on the front door. Through bleary eyes, she was shocked to see a monster of a man standing on the porch. Had to be 6'6 and 270 pounds. He was completely bald but sported a full black beard. He was dressed up like a priest.

"Hello, I am Father Jonathan. Is ZZ in?"

"You bet your ass he is. I will get him."

Stephanie turned and screamed, "ZZ, there is the biggest fucking priest I have ever seen here to see you."

I happened to be coming down the steps and got a monster grin on my face. "Hello Father, sorry for the mouth on my sister. Maybe you can make time later to hear her confession."

Stephanie's face turned bright red as the priest grabbed her hand.

"Stephanie, I have heard so much about you. Your brother thinks you are the most amazing person he ever met. He also has problems with potty mouth, so don't you worry about going to confession," he proclaimed as he kissed her hand.

Just then, Mom ran into the room. She grabbed and hugged Father Jonathan. "Father, it is so good to see you again. I wasn't expecting you, but I hope you can stay for dinner."

I interrupted her, "I hope he can stay longer."

Father Jonathan nodded but added, "The bishop is pretty pissed off," as he removed his collar.

Stephanie looked like she was about to pass out. Mom looked plain shocked. Before Father Jonathan could explain, the sound of a helicopter landing very close to the house made everyone scurry to the porch.

On the front lawn, a pink helicopter with red lips painted on both sides was landing. Grass and yard debris were propelled onto the porch by the wash from the rotors. A few minutes later, the engine stopped, and the door opened. Out popped the cosmetic diva, Azquela Huggins, CEO of Exquisite Evolutions. That was a start-up cosmetics and beauty treatment company. Her current net worth was a couple of a hundred million. She was tall, about six feet. She was not skinny, nor portly, but almost perfectly proportioned. Her black skin was radiant. Her hair was medium length. Not one hair was out of place. Her makeup was tasteful and fully complementary to her features—as you would expect.

She walked to the porch and gave me a big hug and kiss. "ZZ, it's been too long."

"Yes, it has," I replied. I then introduced her to Mom and Stephanie.

"How many guys did you have to blow to get that chopper?" Stephanie inquired,

"Stephanie," Azquela said softly. "I bought that helicopter with money I made in my business. I owe no one anything. Except your brother, Father Jonathan, and this guy coming in now."

Just then, a black limo pulled into the driveway. Out of a back door popped a fireplug of a guy. He was about 5'7 and weighed 200 pounds. Not an inch of fat on his body. He had dark black glasses, dark wavy hair, and a size seventy-nine neck. Running up the steps, he picked Azquela off the ground and twirled her in a circle.

"Boom, boom, boom, nice to see you, sweet cheeks," he said as he kissed her cheek and pinched her ass.

"Good to see you too, Joe," laughed Azquela.

Joe, a.k.a. Guiseppe Crinelli, was the CEO of Crinelli Construction. He was also the grandson of Aldo Crinelli. Aldo was, a.k.a. Razor, a noted gangster. Joe had three bouquets of roses. He gave the first to Mom with a big kiss.

"Hi Mom, nice to be back home."

He gave the next one to Azquela. He never called her that. He had nicknamed her Azzie and that is what most of us called her. "These are nowhere near as beautiful as you, but please accept them."

He then walked over to Stephanie, who, believe it or not, looked a little intimidated. "You must be Stephanie?"

"Fucking A," Stephanie said.

"Well Stephanie, I have these flowers for you. Not only are you as beautiful as ZZ told me, but you tear me up!"

Stephanie took the flowers and gave him a big hug.

Mom invited everyone into the house. "Let me get dinner on. There has to be something big brewing, and I sense that we will need plenty of food to digest all of it."

"Can I get anyone a drink?" I offered.

We had a couple drinks as Mom got dinner ready with Stephanie's help. It was a beautiful spread, considering she had little notice. When she called, we filed into the dining room and sat down. I grabbed a hot dinner roll, and Azzie smacked my fingers.

"How about we pray, you heathen." Azzie giggled. She liked to tease.

Father Jonathon took the cue and stood up.

"Please bow your heads. Dear Father, we thank you for a great meal and great company. We thank you for sparing our lives when we were so young and foolish." (My mother looked up with a quizzical expression on her face but said nothing.) "We thank you for reuniting us to help our friend. Please give us the strength and courage to do whatever is right to allow us all to continue in our service to you."

"Amen," resounded from all sitting at the table.

After the dishes had been cleared and the coffee served, I began the explanation to Mom and Stephanie about our little group.

"When we were roommates at Rutgers, we had become good friends. Unfortunately, like many kids, we got crazy. Long story short, we got hooked on drugs. Heroin, in particular. None of us ever would have injected it, but around the time we were in college, it became cheap and stronger. We all got hooked snorting the stuff, and from there, we moved to injecting."

I looked at my mother, who had tears in her eyes. I was telling her something she never knew.

Stephanie looked as dejected as I had ever seen her. She then screamed out, "You were a fucking junkie?"

"Yes Stephanie," replied Father Jonathan. "We were all junkies. Please let ZZ finish, and then you can judge us."

I continued. "One night, late in the second semester of our freshman year, we scored what we thought was some really good stuff. The four of us got together to party. Azzie, Father Jonathan, and Joe shot up. I was ready to when there was a knock on the door. I answered it. It was another junkie we knew who wanted to borrow some stuff. I turned him away and returned to the living room to find that all three of my friends were not breathing. They were blue and dying. What little I knew from being a junkie told me that I had about three to four minutes before they would suffer brain damage."

"Did you give them Narcan?" asked Mom.

"Well Mom, it was only used in hospitals then, and it had to been injected intravenously. It was not available for public use, and as a nasal spray as it is now."

Azzie stood up and finished the story. "ZZ ran from person to person giving us two breaths. He did this for fifteen minutes until the medics arrived. As you can see, we all survived. We had only ZZ and God to thank. We were all dead without their intervention. When we were all resuscitated and reunited in the ER, we made a pact. We would go to rehab, and we would never do drugs again. We commemorated the day with a solemn promise to never forget that dying was easy. It didn't take a whole hell of a lot of effort to shoot up that day and begin our journey to hell. Had there not been a knock on the door, ZZ would have been with us in route to destination Gehenna. God spared us for a purpose. None of us knows what that was, but there certainly was one. But we all knew that living would be difficult. Transforming from four addicts to clean, successful human beings was a treacherous road. 'Dying Was Easy' became our battle cry when any of us were tempted to use again. We texted the magic words, and the gang showed up. We had plenty of temptation, but no one ever used again. When we finally were able to look our addiction in the rear-view mirror, we kept the battle cry to be used when any of us needed urgent help. Two days ago, ZZ sounded the alarm, and here we are."

"And we aren't going anywhere until the f'ing problem is fixed," said Father Jonathan.

"Are you sure a priest should be using such language?" retorted Joe.

"Hey fireplug, you can wash my mouth out if you want. Oh yah, you can't reach that high," added Father Jonathan with a grin. "I am not a priest until this is over." He raised his fist and screamed, "Dying Was Easy. I may not be going back anyway. The bishop is short of priests and did not want to grant me a leave."

"So how did you get here?" I asked.

"I told him I had made a commitment. I have nothing more to say about it."

I stood. "Mom, Stephanie, the purpose of this reunion is to save Always Hope, the farm, and The Always Hope School. I thought I had

a handle on it until the medical staff suspended me. At that point, I knew
I needed help, and I knew the only place I could go to get it."

CHAPTER 30

Fired Up Farms
1745 July 17

Azzie had gone to her room and retrieved an easel with large sheets of white paper attached. She returned, set up the easel, and opened a felt tip pen.

"Let's get to it," she said.

I laid out the facts as I knew them to the group. Starting with Carl's accident and the financial mess that I found here. I filled them in on the demands of the creditors, and the deal that I made to keep us floating until Millions Week concluded. I then informed them that I had gone back to racing and was racing as much as possible in addition to working in the ER.

"That was until I was suspended from the hospital medical staff on some trumped-up charges. At 9 AM today, that suspension was reported to the state board of medicine. My medical license is now suspended, and my harness licenses are also suspended. But if I appeal the medical suspension, I can drive until it is adjudicated. Provided the appeal is scheduled and concluded within thirty days."

Azzie had made a separate page for each problem. She took copious notes.

I continued, "We have six weeks to come up with the money. If we don't, the horse, the farm, and school are done."

Azzie cleared her throat. "ZZ, you know I normally would have the ability to write you a considerable check. But we have an IPO (Initial Public Stock Offering) coming up and I cannot make any loans or move the kind of funds you need. I am so sorry."

"Hey Azzie, you know I would never ask you to do that. If you did, I would have a hard time accepting it. But I do appreciate the offer."

Joe looked confused. "I don't understand what the medical staff stuff has to do with harness racing."

I took a few minutes to explain NJ SB 12.74 to the group.

Father Jonathan inquired, "When is the appeal?"

"I don't know for sure, but I heard a rumor from a reliable source that it was going to be scheduled for five weeks from now. That's a week after Millions Week. Because that appeal is more than thirty days from the hearing, the suspensions would remain in effect. I wouldn't be able to drive. Worse yet, none of our horses could race. We could never make the nut we have to come up with."

Joe stood. "I smell a pile of shit here. First, Carl goes to prison. Financial bedlam ensues. While you are trying to solve the problem, you get suspended. I want to know a lot more. But before we get too far into this, I'd like more details about your father's conviction."

"OK, but why?"

"Well, it seems to me to be the incident that started the avalanche. Was it real, or was he set up?"

Mom added, "You can also look at the fact that for the past three years, our racing luck got worse, just as Supreme Stables took off. Four years ago, they were small potatoes. Now they are the dominant force in harness racing. There are many on the backside who think they cheat, but they have never been caught."

Father Jonathan inquired about the medical license suspension. I explained about the night in question and how what I thought was a great practice of EM had been turned into something the medical staff likened to a publicity stunt. I explained the accident, the relationship with Hofucker and Marilyn, and my interaction with Buster. I was interrupted by Joe, who was laughing.

"Still with the nicknames, huh? Buster Hyman, that's a classic."

My face was a little red, being in front of my mom and all. But I covered the events of the night and the sham of a hearing that I faced. It was clear to all that I had been railroaded.

Azzie went into overdrive and quickly came up with three separate goals and three teams. She presented her ideas to the group.

"Group one will work on reinstating ZZ's medical license. I will take the lead on this with ZZ. I do have some discretionary funds that I can appropriate without anyone being the wiser. We need the best help we can get, and we need it fast. Group two will investigate matters at the track. That will include the rapid rise of Supreme Stables and the decline of Fired Up Farms. Their second mission will be to engineer the winnings of $5 million in purses and gambling money by the end of Millions Week. Mom, you, Stephanie, and Father Jonathan will manage that with help from ZZ when available."

"We can also use the services of Pisscatcher, Johnson Stevens," I offered, "He knows a lot about the inner workings of the track."

Azzie wrote his name on the sheet. "Pisscatcher is added to the lineup."

"Group three is a group of one. Joe, you don't need a group. You are soooo resourceful."

"Keep slinging it Azzie, I might even buy it," laughed Joe.

"Joe, your mission is to probe Carl Zander's accident. Was it fully investigated? Are there any pieces missing? I agree with you that it seems like all hell broke loose after his conviction. I find that way too convenient for those who want the farm. While you are at it, can you find out any more about the creditors? Are they shills for the real person or persons behind this?"

"Aye aye, Captain Azzie!" Joe said after saluting her.

The wheels were in motion.

CHAPTER 31

Krenshaw Police Headquarters
0945 July 18

"Mr. Crinelli, exactly why in the hell should I help you?" laughed the police chief.

"Because it's the right thing to do."

"But you are a mafia don, are you not?"

"No, not me. My family might have been mixed up at one time, but I run a legitimate construction business."

"Are there any legitimate construction companies?"

"Very funny, but pretty accurate. Anyway, can you help me with the Carl Zander case?"

"Can't you get the court records?" The chief leaned back in his chair.

"I have them. Unfortunately, they are very spotty because he never mounted a defense. He plead and went away."

"What do you need to know?"

"Did he do it?" Joe placed both hands on the front of the chief's desk and looked him in the eye.

"Of course he did, why would he have plead guilty if he didn't?"

"Was there significant evidence?"

"Oh wow. Yeah, there was irrefutable evidence that he was drinking heavily at the Daily Double. He and the deceased were shit-faced. The bartender took Carl's keys, as he usually did when Carl had a snoot full and called them a cab. Carl and the deceased snuck out the back and used a spare key that Carl had in a compartment in the back of the truck. They took off down the road at a high rate of speed, and Carl hit dead on into a tree. The deceased was ejected and died on impact. Carl was trapped in the driver's seat. He was in critical condition but survived, as you know."

"What was his blood alcohol?"

"It was 0.260."

"Any drugs?"

"No."

"Wow, pretty open and shut." Joe searched for another question to ask but came up empty.

"Yeah, the state police reconstructed the accident and came to the same conclusions we did."

"Thanks, I owe you one."

"I am going to take you up on that. Could you have a talk with ZZ?" the chief inquired.

"About what?"

"Well, his attitude for one thing. He spent some time in that holding cell the other night," the chief said, pointing to the other side of the room," because he caused a ruckus at Supreme Medical Center. One of my deputies said he was out of control on at least one previous occasion there."

Joe stood, put both of his hands on the chief's desk, and looked him straight in the eye. "Chief, I thank you for the courtesies you have shown me today. I can assure you of two things. The first is that if ZZ caused a ruckus, he was provoked. The second is that ZZ's friends, including yours truly, smell something fishy going on in this town. We plan on finding the source of that odor and taking care of it."

"Don't get on the wrong side of the law," cautioned the chief.

"I would never think of it." Joe smiled as he offered his hand to the chief.

1300 Fired Up Farms

In between a myriad of calls from investors and brokers, Azzie found time to place several phone calls. She got the same name from three attorneys she trusted—Samuel Issacs. He was the best of the best when it came to medical staff disciplinary defense. Unfortunately, she could not reach Attorney Issacs until Monday. He apparently was out of town. Azzie tried her best to get a call to him today, but she struck out.

1700 Miracle Mile Racetrack and Casino

I dropped Father Jonathan off about two blocks from the track. The group had felt that it would not be wise for anyone to connect me with Father Jonathan as he pursued his undercover role.

I went to the judge's area to see about my license. I took the breathalyzer and passed it, only to learn that I was fined $250 for being late. Then, they told me that my harness licenses were suspended. So, if I was already suspended, why did I have to take the breathalyzer? They said I should have asked about my license before taking the tube. What a crock of shit. Was there any ruling body that I got along with?

Father Jonathan, now known as Little John, made his way to the licensing offices. $50 later, he brought his groom's license up to date. He inquired if any stables were hiring, to which the clerk laughed.

"They all are. The pay is shitty, and the work sucks, but they are hiring. Supreme Stables pays a little more than others, but they are real pricks to work for. Good luck," he said as he handed Little John his license.

Little John found his way to the Supreme Barn and was hired immediately. Luckily, Little John had experience. He had worked for a small stable in Maine. He was to show up at the barn at 6 AM and be ready to work.

His best chance to learn anything about Supreme Stables was dependent upon no one figuring out that he was working with us. That ruled out his staying at our farm. He was able to secure a small room in the groom's quarters for a rate of $100 a week plus a security deposit.

It was hard to keep my concentration on my drive back to the farm. I was going over everything in my head, and all I got was one hell of a headache.

CHAPTER 32

Fired Up Farms
0900 July 21

"Mr. Issacs, this is Azquela Huggins calling. I was hoping to engage your services on behalf of a friend, Dr. Zachary Zander."

"Ms. Huggins, I am sorry, but I am going to have to decline. I simply have too many active cases. I cannot, in all honesty, take on another client."

"Mr. Issacs, is there any way that I can get you to reconsider? My friend has been wrongfully accused of several issues. His career and livelihood rest in the balance. We are willing to pay a premium retainer to secure your services."

"I really could use the premium retainer, but I just cannot take on another case. I pride myself in a very thorough representation of my clients. At this point I am just barely able to service the ones I have. Unfortunately, I have three cases coming to a head in the next few weeks. I am sorry."

"Can you suggest someone else? With your reputation, I am sure my friend will accept your recommendation."

Issacs looked up to his ceiling and let out a loud sigh.

"I can't believe I am doing this, but I can recommend Daniel Santucci. He and I actually hate each other. But he is truly knowledgeable and does not mind getting his hands dirty, if you know what I mean. He is a small player in our field, but he might have a future."

Supreme Stables, 0900

Father Jonathan had been accepted into Supreme Stables. After a few days, they actually loved him. He worked hard and kept his mouth shut. He asked no questions.

Carlton Hennessey, the head trainer for Supreme Stables, stopped at the stall where Little John was working. "Where did you work before this? You are quite good."

"I worked for a small stable in Maine when I was in high school."

"That was a few years ago. What have you been doing since?" Hennessey asked.

"Nothing that would interest you."

"Try me," Hennessey pressed the issue.

"Look, I do not know if you noticed but you were not the only stable hiring. I do not like to discuss my past, and it's none of your damn business. So, forget the inquisition, or I am moving on."

"Ho! Sorry. You have a hair trigger huh?"

"I do my job and don't bother anyone or anything, take it or leave it."

"Well, we'll take it. Thanks for the help. Can you get the big mare ready next?"

"Sure."

Office of Daniel Santucci Esq. PC.

Clarkstown, NJ 1030

"Azzie Huggins?" Daniel Santucci said as he looked at her business card.

"Yes, I am the CEO of Exquisite Evolutions."

"Holy moly, my wife uses your stuff. Costs me a fortune."

"Maybe you can make a little back."

"Who did you say referred you?" Dan asked as he continued to stare at Azzie's business card.

"Sam Issacs."

"Well, I can't help you," he said as he handed Azzie back her card.

"Why not?" Azzie replied. She set the card on his desk and helped herself to a seat. Even though no one had invited her to sit.

"Anyone that Sam would send me must be a big pain in the ass with an unwinnable case. Sam and I do not get along," Dan said as he scanned his desk calendar, attempting to see what was up for the day. He avoided eye contact with Azzie.

"He mentioned that. I quote, He and I hate each other, but he is extremely knowledgeable, and he doesn't mind getting his hands dirty if you know what I mean." Azzie accidentally left out the part about Dan being a small player in the field.

"He said that?"

"Yes. I got the impression that he thought you were almost as good as he was. From what I hear, he thinks he is the best attorney ever created." Azzie had never heard that, but she was trying to make a sale, and all was fair.

"That's Sam. I never thought he had any respect for me. Interesting. Who is your client, and where does he work?"

"Zachary Zander is an ER doctor at Supreme Medical."

"AHH interesting."

"Why is that?"

"Well, I can never prove it, but that place appears to be the most crooked hospital I have ever seen. I have represented two physicians removed from staff there."

"How did those cases turn out?"

"Lost the first and struck a deal in the second, but the physician still had to leave town. I was able to spare any restrictions on his license, and he is doing well in his new location."

"Sounds like no wins, one loss and one tie to me. Not too impressive." Azzie knew she had to bruise his ego a little to get him interested.

"Yeah, not up to my normal successful stats, but things there are different."

Azzie went on to explain about my relation to Fired Up Stables and our current financial plight. She told him what she knew about the medical staff issues and my past stellar records in both harness racing and medicine. She might have embellished those a trifle.

"Look, Dr. Zander needs these charges dropped and his license reinstated in the next three weeks. Because of the NJ law, his medical license suspension caused a suspension of his harness owner's, trainer's, and driver's licenses on July 17."

"SB 12.74 rears its ugly head," Dan uttered as he shook his.

"Dr. Zander's financial deadlines can only be met if he is able to drive at the Millions Mile week and race his horses there. So, his medical license has to be restored before then."

"Wow. A tough, high-profile case, with a short deadline. Sorry, but that's a non-starter for me. Most of these cases takes months. I don't want another loss on my record," Dan said as he opened his briefcase and withdrew some papers.

"High profile?" Azzie inquired.

"Everyone in the state who has anything to do with medical staff privileges and hospital disciplinary actions knows about it. Not the details, just the short strokes. The rumor is that some hot shit ER doc did a C-section on a pregnant trauma victim who should have been sent to a trauma center. For what it's worth, the word on the street is that this kid is a cocky bastard who got way over his skis, if you know what I mean."

Azzie stood and interrupted Dan.

"Look, I am the CEO of a very successful company. I know talent when I see it, and I also know Dr. Zander. For what it's worth (she pantomimed Dan's voice), I know he would never 'hot dog' with someone's life. He risks his life on the racetrack every night, but when it comes to his patients, he is first rate. I also get the sense that you have a feeling that things at Supreme Medical may not be totally on the up and up. I also get the feeling that you are an up-and-coming hot shit lawyer who sometimes leans a little far over on his skis. I think you are the perfect person for this case, and I know that winning this case could cement your future in the business."

"Losing it could have the opposite effect," Dan said in a matter-of-fact tone.

"There are no guarantees in life. Will you take it?"

"I must admit that I am intrigued. But let us put all the cards on the table. Unfortunately, I would respectfully have to ask for an exceptionally large fee. You see, with the short time frame, I will have to broom all my other cases away. That will cost me significant income and might cost me a client or two. I hate to be such a mercenary, but my wife and I are building a new house. Every night, she comes up with some addition or change that increases the cost exponentially. My builder just licks his chops and puts his hand out."

"Do you mind if I put something on the table?" Azzie asked.

Before Dan could answer, Azzie lifted a hot pink briefcase with her trademark lips onto the desk. She opened it and turned it to face the shocked attorney.

"You are looking at $100,000 in Bitcoin. Untraceable. You can consider this your retainer if you accept. There will be no receipts or records of this. You will bill me for reasonable charges for your services from here on out. If you walk away from the case, I could never prove that I gave you this. But I am a good judge of people. I know you won't do that."

"I am an officer of the court. I cannot accept money that is untraceable and unreported," Dan said without taking his eyes off the briefcase.

"Good," replied Azzie as she stood up and walked to the door. "You never took any money, and I misplace that briefcase all the time."

She didn't wait for Dan to say another word. She handed him a piece of paper with the address to the farm.

"Come to the farm tomorrow at 9 AM, and we will get you up to speed. If you are as good as Issacs said, I might even arrange for a friend to meet with your contractor to work out reasonable prices for your wife's additions. See you tomorrow."

CHAPTER 33

Fired Up Farms
0830 July 22

Things started early at the farm. Mom had breakfast on the table at 5 AM. Soon thereafter she and Stephanie had departed for the racetrack. After Joe made some phone calls, he joined me for a cup of coffee.

"So, you didn't get much from the police?" I inquired.

"Less than nothing. They did a rapid investigation once it was known that Carl wanted to make a quick plea. What they turned up supported the charges. The case was put to bed easily."

"Do you want to work on something else? I can have you dig around at the hospital."

"No, not yet. I still want to trace a few of Carl's steps and be sure that I find nothing out of line. His accident was still way too convenient for my liking. The pieces fit together too nicely. Cases aren't normally like that. It reminds me of when I suspect theft in my business. At first glance, things look copasetic, and the stories always add up. When they add up too perfectly my bullshit detector goes off. Then I peel the onion. My BS detector is not red yet, but it isn't green either, so I think I will dig a little more. That bartender Jerome strikes me as a liar. The one waitress I talked to was an airhead. But the waitress who may have had the most contact with Carl wasn't there. She is due to work tomorrow and I plan to interview her. Did you know that by some coincidence, the security camera covering the back lot where Carl parked was broken for about a month before the accident? Jerome claimed he didn't have enough cash to fix it."

"You are a great friend," I said as I stood.

"See you tonight!" Joe yelled as he walked out the door.

Azzie and I reviewed the financial picture, which was bleak. We were going to have to net $5 million during Millions Week to squeak by. Then Azzie delivered the knockout punch.

"You know that even if we pull this off, you have only about three or four months before the bills pile up again. You can easily run the racing operation, but the school is going to bury you."

"I know you are right, but for some stupid reason, I think once we get past Millions Week, we will work something out." I smiled.

"With a major shit storm flying around you, you are a wild optimist?"

"Yeah, must have been that kick in the head." I pointed at my scar.

The doorbell rang. I looked out the window at a small man in a suit. Couldn't have been more than 5' 2", and I doubted if he weighed more than 95 pounds. He looked like a thoroughbred jockey in a suit. He had curly hair and wire-rimmed glasses. His necktie was bright blue and clashed with his suit.

"Hello, I am Daniel Santucci. Is Dr. Zander at home?"

"Dr. Zander is taking a shit, but ZZ is here." I laughed and grabbed his hand.

Azzie ran past me and grabbed Santucci's other hand, causing him to drop his briefcase. "Thank you so much for coming."

"I like a good challenge," he said as she walked him into the house.

"Coffee anyone?" I was getting good at making coffee. Good thing, I might be working at Starbucks when this is all over.

"Better get them all around ZZ, this will take a while," Azzie screamed as I exited toward the kitchen.

As I brought the coffee, Santucci asked, "I take it you prefer ZZ to Dr. Zander?"

"Yeah, oh sorry about the introduction. I was expecting some asshole from Supreme Medical any minute, and I thought you might be him."

"No need to apologize. For what this is about to cost you, I will call you anything you want. Let us get down to business. Here is a list of my fees. I expect payment whether you win or lose. In the contract, you will see that I have the right to use consultants, detectives, police contacts, etc., at my discretion, and at your expense. Are you both ok with this?"

Azzie stood and said, "I personally guarantee that you will be pleased with the compensation. I will be happy to sign the agreement, promissory note, or whatever you require. All I expect for my money is the most thorough defense of a client that you have ever mounted. If you uncover a conspiracy to hurt ZZ, I would appreciate the total legal destruction of anyone involved."

"Azzie, I can't!" I protested vehemently.

"You sounded the warning, and you will do what the team feels is necessary," Azzie added curtly.

"Mr. Santucci, you should know by now, if you don't already, that no one messes with Azzie when she is on a mission," I offered.

Dan nodded. "Good, let's get to work. Please tell me as much as you can, and in as much detail as you can, about the hearing and that night in the ER."

"Shouldn't there be transcripts?" Azzie asked.

"Ideally yes, but realistically no. There may be a few cryptic and misleading notes, but no transcripts. Medical staffs are notorious for having bland and unhelpful meeting minutes."

I described the night in question and the hearing as best as I could. It took well over an hour and a half. I was a little annoyed that Santucci never took a single note. I was expecting him to write half a book and then pepper me with questions about my medical decisions. But that was not what I got.

"Was there anyone in particular on the committee after you?"

"No, they were all like sharks after a fresh meal."

"They found you guilty on six charges, is that correct?"

"Yes sir," I answered without looking up.

Dan ran down the list to be sure he had it right. Suddenly, it hit me. This dude never took a note, but he just recited the charges almost verbatim. Some kind of photographic memory I reckon. I was impressed.

Dan summed things up. "The allegations of inappropriate death of Cynthia Walker, inappropriate C-section, and loss of donated organs are all clinical matters. We will need some expert witnesses to assist us in defending those. The supposed HIPPA violation is total crap, and I expect they will agree to drop that in return for some concession on our part. It does appear that you did exhibit inappropriate behavior at both medical staff meetings. You conceded that in the trial, so we can't do anything about that. Can I ask why you did not report the incident of moral turpitude as was required by the rules and regulations?"

"Counselor, to be totally honest, I never read the bylaws, rules, and regulations. As a locum's physician, I work in about ten different hospitals a year. Even if I had horrible insomnia, I could never read them all. So, although I found the behavior unacceptable, I didn't know that reporting was required. I would have, had it occurred again. I believe in second chances."

"I understand. No one reads the bylaws, rules, and regulations. You are not unique. It's job security to me. They mean nothing until they mean something, and now for you, they mean everything. The rules and regulations did require you to report moral turpitude."

"How can I report something if I don't even know what the hell it means?"

Dan grinned, "Conduct that is believed to be contrary to community standards of honesty, good morals, or justice."

"Counselor, it may shock you, but many an orgasm has been experienced in ERs around the country."

"That doesn't surprise me." He sipped his coffee and thought for a few seconds. "Here's how I think they will play this. They pump up the two charges you are guilty of as much as they can. They hope to taint the panel into thinking you are a loose cannon. Then they run the other charges by quickly and hope that either the panel buys the whole enchilada, or you lose your cool and walk out. Then they win by default."

"How do we proceed?" I was cautiously optimistic.

"You must stay out of the hospital. If you get calls from anyone on the staff or any correspondence, do not respond. Route everything through me or Azzie. Do not share our proposed defense with anyone, and I mean anyone. You, Azzie, and I are the only ones to discuss this. I know you trust your family and friends, but they might accidentally say the wrong thing to the wrong person. We have little margin for error here."

"OK I understand."

"We may need some information from the hospital medical staff personnel. Have you managed to piss them off too, or can I expect some cooperation?"

"You can trust Juicy Lucy but stay away from Not Too Juicy Lucy."

"Run that by me again?" Dan had a quizzical look on his face.

I explained, "both the medical staff secretary and her assistant are named Lucy. I nicknamed the assistant Juicy Lucy. She is a friend. Her boss is Not Too Juicy Lucy, and she does hate me."

Azzie laughed, "Juicy Lucy? ZZ you are nuts!"

Dan was straight-faced. "Alright, at least we know who to talk with and who not to. Azzie, can you call and try to get an idea of when the appeal is scheduled for?"

"I can do that," I offered.

Dan waved me off, "I'd rather you and I finish our discussion. Was the doctor who was injured really named Hofucker?"

"His name is Hofecker, I call him Hofucker."

"Thanks, I don't want to make that mistake during the appeal."

"Did I mention that Hofucker is the CEO's son?" I was sure that I hadn't.

I then shared with Santucci the interaction I had with Hofecker II on my first night on duty, and the allegation of Medicare fraud.

"Well ZZ, you do know how to push people's buttons don't you?" He laughed.

In the corner of the room, Azzie placed her phone call.

"Supreme Medical, Medical Staff Office, Lucy speaking," said the voice on the other end of the phone.

Azzie wasn't sure how to determine if this was the Lucy who was the friend or foe. "I am calling on behalf of Dr. Zander. He told me that you might be able to assist me in his defense."

"If you are a friend of Dr. Zander, then you know his nickname for me. What is it?"

Azzie blushed, "Juicy Lucy?"

"Ah, very good. He cracks me up with his nicknames. My boss is an old wombat, and his name for her is perfect. What can I do for you? Be quick, as I expect Not Too Juicy Lucy to return at any moment."

Azzie asked if it was known when the appeal was scheduled for.

"September 15th."

Azzie read her a list of items that might help Dan and gave her Dan's email address.

Lucy read them back and added, "Some of those items are confidential to the hospital. I could lose my job if I am caught."

Azzie immediately retorted, "Then don't get caught. I assure you Dan knows how to use information without divulging its source."

"Ok, tell that ZZ that I expect a visit from Mr. G before my wedding."

"Ahhh," Azzie stuttered because she wasn't sure what to say except "OK and thanks."

Azzie returned as Dan was making a few notes.

He finished and addressed her. "Azzie, as I told you, we will have to spend some money, and due to our time constraints, we can't afford to shop around. I will need experts in the areas of Ob-Gyn, and organ transplant, in addition to an ER physician. The kind of folks I am thinking about will run you $20,000 each."

"No problem, get the best, and ZZ, don't even start. Because of you, I am above the grass instead of below it, and doing quite well. Plus, it will be great to watch when Mr. Santucci destroys those pricks."

"Everyone, please call me Dan."

Just then, there was a knock on the door. Azzie answered it, and there in the doorway stood Deputy Taser. Holy shit, they were coming to arrest me for something. Azzie signed a slip of paper, and Deputy Taser handed her an envelope. I flipped him the bird (ok so the door was already closed but I still flipped it). Azzie handed the envelope to me. It was from Supreme Medical. I quickly opened and read it.

As Azzie had told us the appeal was scheduled for September 15th. That was about two weeks too late to save my licenses.

"Are we screwed or what?" I sighed.

"Or what," Dan replied. "We are never screwed until I say so. Let me see the notice."

The appeal was scheduled for September 15th, and they were using Eiton Shapiro again as a hearing officer. Dan mentioned that he had run into him during his previous interactions with Supreme Medical. He further informed us that he thought Shapiro was competent but not unbeatable.

I objected. "That prick Eat A Ton ran the first hearing. He's the bastard that got Martines and I locked up. He is completely biased. Can't we get someone else?" I really didn't want to see that dude again.

Dan grinned, "You are going to get me in trouble with your nicknames. I could easily slip up. I know the next time I look at him, I will be thinking, 'Eat A Ton'. I just hope I don't say it!" He continued, "The hospital gets to pick the hearing officer. But don't be too concerned. Shapiro is an arrogant ass. The last time I faced him, I was a little timid. I like going up against a known entity. I will be ready for him this time."

Two seconds later, his cell phone appeared in his hand out of nowhere. It was like watching a gunslinger draw. He began breathing fire and spitting orders into the phone.

"Prepare a request for an emergency injunction hearing to occur this week. Zander case, reasons for hearing will be two: 1. Requesting emergency relief for timing of appeal of suspension of medical staff privileges. Appeal time frame is too long to prevent automatic suspension of Dr. Zander's other licenses. 2. Requesting emergency relief requiring Supreme Medical to use a hearing panel consisting of at least one peer to the defendant as opposed to the use of a hearing officer as they have proposed. I will be back in the office in an hour. I want to file this before 3 PM. Get a draft ready. Thanks."

Azzie looked calm, but I was shitting bricks. She asked Dan, "Is there anything else we can tell you, or help you with?"

Dan was packing his stuff up, and I think he was already standing, but with his stature problem, that was hard to tell.

"We will get a hearing this week, my guess is it will be Friday. Keep an eye on your emails. I tend to do a lot of work via email. I will be in touch."

In less than fifteen seconds, he was out the door.

"Oh, by the way ZZ, Juicy Lucy said to tell you that she is expecting a visit from Mr. G before her wedding," Azzie giggled.

It was one of the few times in my life that I didn't know what to say.

CHAPTER 34

Daily Double Bar
1100 July 23

Joe's phone rang as he arrived in the parking lot of the Daily Double Bar. By the "Godfather" theme ringtone he knew right away who was calling, but he answered in his normal fashion anyway.

"Hello, what the hell do you want?" he bellowed into the car speaker.

"You tear me up when you answer the phone like that Guiseppe." It was Aldo Crinelli, a.k.a. Razor.

"Sorry grandpa, I get a lot of calls from assholes and telemarketers."

"Me too, pricks. Anyway, I got the info that you requested."

"Thanks grandpa, tell me."

"Your bartender is a squirrel. A squirrel that likes to bet on baseball and basketball. The problem is that he is not particularly good at it. My contacts say he got into his book for around $50K."

"Wow, that really helps, anything else?"

"As a matter of fact, there is. He was paying five percent vigorish per week. But most weeks he couldn't come up with the full vig. As you know any shortfall got added to the principal."

"So, they were burying the bastard with the vig."

"Yeah, and then they shut off his betting, so he had no way to come up with the cash. The rumor was that they were going after the bar. Then bammo, out of the blue, he pays off half the balance about four months ago. From that point on he made every vig payment. A couple months ago, he paid off the full balance."

"So, the squirrel came into some cash?"

"He claimed that he made a big score on a three-way parlay. But that doesn't wash for two reasons. First and foremost, he was shut off. No one would take his action, and the legal sports books don't offer credit. Second, he said it was one parlay. Why pay off half the balance and continue to pay vig when you can afford to pay it all off?"

"Sounds like he got paid one half up front for something, and the second half when the job was done."

"Bingo!"

"Thanks grandpa, this really helps."

"Anything for ZZ. That kid saved your life. I will never forget it. Plus, I want to be able to bet him in the Millions. You will get me some inside information, won't you?"

"Grandpa!" Joe protested.

He just laughed and hung up.

It was about 11 AM when Joe walked in and saw Jerome, the squirrel, behind the bar washing some glasses.

"What can I get you?" the squirrel asked.

"Is Denise working today?" Joe inquired.

"Talk to her on her own time, not mine. If you want a drink, order it. If not, shove off. I told you everything I know the other day."

Joe leaned over the bar and grabbed Jerome by his black tie.

"Look buddy, I don't think I care for your attitude. I am going to talk to Denise whether you like it or not. The only thing in question here is whether I beat the shit out of you first. Lucky for you I am short of time today."

Joe released the tie, threw $20 on the bar, and said, "That's more than you pay her in an hour. I don't think I will need her that long. Keep the change. Maybe you can parlay that into a fortune. You are the parlay king are you not?"

The squirrel said nothing but looked shocked. He picked up the money and went back to washing glasses as Denise came out of the kitchen.

"Are you Denise?"

"Who's asking?"

"I'm Joe Crinelli, a friend of Zachary Zander."

"Oh ZZ, how is he? He hasn't been in for a while."

"Can we go somewhere to talk?"

"I'm on duty and the damn bartender has it in for me, maybe some other time."

"I just paid for you to take an hour off, do you mind going to my car?"

"Hey, I don't do that shit."

"Sorry, I just want conversation. That's all. I don't want to do it in here."
Joe handed her a fifty-dollar bill as they walked out behind the bar to his car.

"I hope that creep doesn't have his cameras running." Denise said.

"What creep, what cameras?"

"A few months ago, my boyfriend was on a long trip. He got home early and stopped at the bar. It had been a while, if you know what I mean. On my break, we ended up in the back seat of his car. Two days later the creep that lives over there, (she pointed to a house beyond the back parking lot), met me at my car. He showed me a video of Gus and I going at it. He wanted $500 not to post it on Facebook."

"Did you pay him?"

"No, but Gus paid him a visit. He happened to give Gus the tape for free."

"Oh, it sounds like Gus can be persuasive."

"Yeah, he is an MMA fighter."

"Pummeled his ass, I bet."

"No, Gus isn't like that. The guy was a big MMA fan and Gus gave him an autographed picture and tickets to an upcoming event."

"OK, I am not sure if I believe that, but I wanted to ask you about the night Carl Zander had his accident."

"Anything in particular?"

"No, just anything you recall."

"He and Ken came in to celebrate the birth of Ken's first child. They bought a round of drinks for the house and had a toast. Then they went into the back room to play pool."

"Did you serve them?"

"In a way, I did."

"You are going to have to explain that better, either you did, or you didn't."

"I served them their drinks for the toast, but they used the train for the other drinks."

"Train?"

"Yeah, if you notice, there is a model train that goes from the main bar to the pool room. People get a kick out of ordering from the train. If they are running a tab they put a drink order in the mail car of the train. The train takes it to the server's work area. We, or the bartender process the order and load the drinks on the train. It takes them to the station in the pool room."

"Did Carl and Ken use the train that night?"

"They always did. They both were train nuts, and when they got a little hammered, they liked it even more."

"At the trial, Jerome testified that Carl and Ken had six drinks each. He said they were double scotches. Is that right?"

Denise shrugged her shoulders. "I have no idea. I served them the initial toast and after that, they used the train. Jerome must have filled their orders after the toast. I never saw them after that."

"With six double scotches on board, they had to be pretty wasted. You said that you didn't see them after the toast. Did anyone you know see them?"

"I have no idea."

Joe realized that she had nothing more to offer about their condition, so he changed the line of questioning.

"Speaking of hammered, did Carl hit the booze often?"

"Not too often, once every couple of weeks or so. But when he did, he liked to get a snoot full."

"Did he ever drive home?"

"The night of the wreck."

"Other than that?"

"No, his wife always came to get him."

"Did you see any unusual people in here on the night of the wreck?"

"There are always unusual people in this place, but nothing out of the ordinary that night."

"Anything else about the night stick out?"

"No." She paused. "Wait. That was the night Jerome got sick. Said he had the shits or something and left early. Maggie and I had to serve food, make drinks, and manage the crowd at the bar. It was a big pain in the ass."

"What time did he leave?"

"I am not sure of the time, but I know it was before the accident. I remember asking him about Carl's tab when he was leaving. He told me that he closed it out and had shut them off."

CHAPTER 35

Barn 7

Miracle Mile Racetrack and Casino

1200 July 23

There were five qualifiers scheduled for today. We had only one horse in to qualify, Fired Up Alabama. Stephanie had talked her way into driving in all four other races. Other than at Supreme Stables, she was extremely popular at the track. Why not, she grew up there. These people were her friends and family.

I had my daily conference call with Dan at 2 PM but my morning was free. Luckily, the security guards at the backside gate knew me. I waved and they let me pass. Had they verified my license they would have found out that I had been suspended.

After helping with the morning chores, I assisted Mom and Stephanie with getting Alabama ready. Alabama was making her first start. She had incredible talent but was a head case.

Qualifiers were kind of weird because there were no fans to cheer or jeer. Just five or six horses in a race. The only people potentially paying attention to the races were the drivers in the race, the owners if they were present or watching on the internet, or the grooms if they gave a shit. Plus, there was no one calling the race. Why call a race if no one was listening? There was no money to be won. The only thing the horses had to do was to beat a pretty easy-to-obtain qualifying time, not break, and not make an ass of themselves.

I almost cried as they came out for the first qualifier. Stephanie was driving Burnt Toast. That's not what made me cry. I had never seen Stephanie in her driving colors. They were remarkably like mine. Every little detail was the same, except that instead of 'ZZ' on her back, there was 'SZ.' She had honored me by adopting my colors. She even had on sunglasses with gold lenses. The kind that was standard issue to sheriffs in the deep south. They had been one of my trademarks.

Burnt Toast was a mere mortal horse, a $10,000 claimer. But he was 11 and had become a barn pet. He was coming back from an injury and needed to show that he could race competitively again. His connections were very good friends of Stephanie, and they were delighted for her to qualify him. When the gate pulled away, Stephanie wasted no time. She put Burnt Toast on the front. She backed off the second quarter and let him loose. He won going away. It was a nice drive.

She had a horse shipping in from Pennsylvania in the second qualifier. She tried to leave for the front with her but she got outstepped by Billie Cha-ching. She managed to squeeze herself into the three-hole and ended up finishing second.

In the third race, she got away last and sat patiently there until the ¾ pole where she let the horse loose and won easily. The trainer was ecstatic. He had told her to go to the front. She said the horse didn't feel right behind the gate, so she didn't. As it turns out, the trainer had been convinced that the horse needed to race on the front. Now he knew that she could do it both ways. He slipped Stephanie a $100 bill.

The fourth race was a real bore. She was in the four-hole. She got away fourth and finished fourth. The horse qualified and Stephanie got another drive under her belt. But there would be no mention of this race in the sports pages, or anywhere. It wasn't her fault. The horse was just an average campaigner.

Alabama was in the fifth and last qualifier. There were a number of unknowns in the race in addition to the known horse, Supreme Milkshake. He was three and highly staked. He had never started in a parimutuel race but this was his second qualifier. The Supremes liked to have their horses really tight, (ready to race), when they dropped him in the box. Milkshake was just average in his first qualifier, (even though he won), so they wanted to qualify him again.

Stephanie left out the four-hole and easily got the lead with Alabama. Billie pulled Milkshake to the outside and tried to get to the top. Tried was the operative word. He brushed up quickly, but Stephanie was chilly on the bike. She looked like she was at the farm on a Sunday afternoon. She had Billie parked out. Luckily for Billie, the horse behind Stephanie broke. He got Milkshake to the rail right behind her.

Alabama commanded the lead to the top of the stretch. Billie pulled to the outside as five chosen members of the Autistic Army exploded in a chorus of encouragement for Alabama. I was wrong about no one watching the races. None of our horses raced unless some, or all, of the members of The Army were there. Today there were five along with their handlers and they were animated.

Billie whipped his horse mercilessly as Stephanie just sat still. Around mid-stretch, she flipped her right wrist and Alabama rolled to a three-length victory. As she slowed Alabama down Billie deliberately got close enough to rub wheels to intimidate Stephanie. Stephanie wasn't fazed until she heard the snap. One of Billie's lines had broken. With only one line he had no control of his horse. Milkshake went into high gear without any pressure on his bit. Billie was just a passenger. He had a few options, all bad.

One was to turn around on the bike and jump off. Going about thirty mph jumping onto a limestone surface was usually painful. Two, he could just sit on the bike and hope the horse didn't dump him out before the horse got tired. His third option was to stand up on the bike and leap onto the horse's ass. If he made it that far he could then climb onto the horse's back.

Being a wild man, Billie had decided that he would try to jump on the horse's back. As he prepared to stand up, he saw a blur to his left. It was Alabama with Stephanie driving furiously. Alabama passed them on the left and Stephanie reached up with her right hand and grabbed Milkshake's halter. She gradually slowed Alabama and Milkshake down and pulled them to a stop.

Everyone watching the race or getting their horse ready to go back to the barn had lined up behind the fence. A broken line could be a death sentence. What Stephanie had done was a miracle. Few drivers could pull it off.

Billie jumped from the bike and handed the one rein he had to the groom. He went over to Stephanie and got down on his knees to thank her. He was appreciative but he was also a showboat. I had never seen such a driving feat. Everyone headed back to the barn. No harm no foul.

Deuce was waiting at his barn when Billie returned.

"I I I I go go got got l lu lucky Mr. Hofecker. I I I cou cou cou da da been kil kil killed."

"Look you stuttering imbecile you are through."

"Wha wha why?"

"Because I had the judges convinced that your line broke because the bitch drifted into you after the wire. You were startled and pulled back hard on the reins when it happened. Since it was after the wire the race tape didn't show it. They were prepared to pull her provisional license. But your stunt of kneeling in front of her ruined the whole thing. As soon as the judges saw that they changed their minds. You would never have done that if she almost killed you. Get your ass out of here."

CHAPTER 36

1256 Houston Lane

Krenshaw, NJ

0900 July 24

Joe hoped that the prick was home. This was his third trip to this shithole, and he was hoping it was his last. But more importantly, he was hoping to find the information that he needed. He made his way to the shack whose property bordered the back parking lot of The Daily Double. Two of the windows were covered with plastic. Rusty Christmas ornaments that had been hung years ago were sagging from the roof. Fast food containers lined the sidewalk near an overflowing garbage can. In the evergreens that separated the parking lot from this decrepit abode, Joe noticed a number of small cameras. He knocked on the door.

The door opened slightly, still secured by the chain lock. A small dude covered with bad ink on his face and neck hid behind the crack. Joe counted at least ten visible piercings.

"Who are you, and what do you want?"

"My name is Joe, and I was hoping we could do some business."

"Hey asshole, I don't deal anymore. Ask my parole officer. I am clean. Get the fuck out of here."

"No one wants any drugs. I am interested in conversation, and I like to watch home videos." Joe flashed a roll of one-hundred-dollar bills. "I pay well for particularly good ones."

The piercing poster child focused on the money roll. "Ok then, come on in."

There was more garbage in the living room than what he saw outside. Joe did however notice five flatscreen monitors with live video feeds. It appeared to be various shots of the Daily Double exits and parking lot. On the table were two miniature drones.

"What particular video might you be interested in?"

"Well, I am intrigued by the Daily Double Bar. Such a quaint place."

"As it turns out I might have something to interest you." His outstretched hand was palm up.

Joe put a $100 bill in his palm.

"That's a nice start, what do you want to see?"

"What do you have?"

"These five monitors show what's on the cameras aimed at the Daily Double."

"Why there?"

"Hey man, lots of interesting shit goes down there. Drug deals, prostitution, cheating spouses, etc. You wouldn't believe how many people get interested in their own or significant other's videos."

"I imagine certain videos can be quite valuable."

"Most aren't worth shit, but every now and again I make a score."

Joe went over to the monitor as Piercemaster showed him how he could zoom in and out and get a pretty good view of the back of the bar and the parking lot.

"The bar is ok, but the parking lot is where I get most of my action. Lots of stuff goes down in cars in that parking lot. The camera angles get into most cars without heavy window tint. What I can't see with the fixed cameras, I often pick up with the drones." He pointed to the drones on the table. "I can get them right beside the windows or above the truck beds. Great resolution."

"Do you save any of the videos, or do you record over them?"

"I save about a year's worth in the cloud. If I haven't done anything with it by then I discard them."

Joe stood and slowly peeled off ten one-hundred-dollar bills and placed them on an end table.

"Can you show me all that you have for the evening of April 8th. From 5 PM until midnight will do. That cash is yours for the trouble. If I see anything I like I can get you another $4,000 for a copy."

CHAPTER 37

Municipal Courtroom 3
Krenshaw, NJ
1000 July 25

I sat at the attorney's table on the right side of the courtroom with Azzie and Dan. Azzie and I were nervous. Dan was calm. At the opposition table sat Eat A Ton Shapiro, the attorney for Supreme Medical, Deuce, and Buster.

"Dan," I whispered. "Can I shoot a spitball at their table? I know you won't let me flip them off."

Dan whispered back "ZZ, you know the rules. You don't talk unless I direct you to. You don't react, either positively or negatively, to anything said or done. Agreed?"

"Agreed."

The bailiff announced, "All stand. Municipal court 12-6 now in session. The Honorable Samantha Robinson presiding."

"Mr. Santucci, present your case." The judge wasted no time getting started.

Dan stood and took a moment to readjust his glasses. Then he launched. "Your honor, my client Dr. Zachary Zander is a board-certified emergency physician who also happens to be a world-renowned harness race driver." He paused to let that sink in, and then he continued.

"Dr. Zander has never been suspended or reprimanded by either the medical board or the harness racing commission. However, he recently received a summary suspension of his privileges to practice emergency medicine at Supreme Medical Center. This suspension not only prevents him from practicing medicine, but it also affects his harness racing license due to NJ SB 12.74"

"And your point counselor?" queried the judge.

"Your honor, I intend to prove during appeal that my client did not deviate from the standard of emergency care and that his suspension was arbitrary and capricious."

"I object" came a forceful voice from a massively rotund body sitting at the Supreme table. The objector jumped to a standing position. It was hard to believe that 375 pounds of almost pure fat could move that fast. The voice and proposity of adiposity belonged to Eat A Ton, Shapiro.

"State your objection." Judge Robinson demanded.

"The plaintiff in this case had a fair hearing. Based upon his deviation from the standard of care, he was suspended by his peers. There was nothing arbitrary or capricious about the process."

"Mr. Shapiro, you are wound up today, aren't you? I asked Mr. Santucci what his case was. You may not agree with it, but you can't object to his statement. You know better."

"OVERRULED!" The gavel smacked the wooden holder with a loud thud but Judge Robinson was not done. "This is an emergency injunction hearing. Please cut out the usual courtroom garbage. Anyone embellishing, overly objecting, or otherwise lengthening these proceedings unnecessarily will be sorry. Mr. Santucci, proceed."

"Supreme Medical Center has scheduled an appeal of their egregious ruling on September 15. I am sorry judge, please strike egregious."

Judge Robinson nodded with a small smile on her face. Dan continued.

"Supreme Medical has scheduled the appeal on September 15th. That time frame significantly harms my client. NJ SB 12.74 provides that a suspension of one license does not affect other licenses provided an appeal is requested and completed within thirty days. This appeal is scheduled beyond that thirty-day window.

Based upon the current timeframe Dr. Zander would not be permitted to drive, train, or own a harness horse in competition in the state of New Jersey until the appeal is heard. Nor would he be permitted to practice medicine. Based upon what we feel was an unfair trial his ability to earn would be severely affected. To prevent irreparable harm to Dr. Zander we request that the appeal be scheduled within 30 days of the initial hearing."

"Mr. Shapiro?" uttered Judge Robinson.

Eat A Ton stood slowly this time and exhaled loudly. He stroked his beard as he spoke. "Dr. Zander was evaluated with strict adherence to the rules and regulations of Supreme Medical Center. The same rules and regulations he agreed to when he joined the staff. The outcome was not favorable to Dr. Zander, but that has nothing to do with the process. The process was fair."

"Mr. Santucci?" Judge Robinson threw the ball back to Dan.

"We contend that the process was not fair."

Shapiro bellowed, "Do tell, son."

"Ok pops."

Judge Robinson had raised her arm to wrap the gavel. Instead, she got a grin on her face with Dan's retort. She let him continue.

"The process used a hearing officer, in lieu of a hearing panel. The hearing officer was none other than Mr. Shapiro. Mr. Shapiro is not a physician, and therefore not a peer of the physician being investigated."

Shapiro shook his head. "The by-laws allow for that option."

Santucci agreed. "Yes, they do. Your honor, those by-laws are flawed."

Robinson looked over her glasses. "Counselor, the by-laws are the by-laws. They are binding to homeowners' associations, country clubs, hospitals, etc. If the investigation met the requirement of the by-laws, then why should the suspension not stand?"

Dan took a moment and looked at his notes. "Your honor, if you will indulge me for five minutes, I believe I can demonstrate why the by-laws are flawed."

"Five minutes maximum Mr. Santucci!"

Dan turned toward Shapiro. "Is Supreme Medical Center accredited by an accrediting body?"

Eat A Ton shot back immediately. "We are fully accredited by the most acknowledged and credible body, The Joint Commission."

"So Supreme Medical Center is required to meet appropriate Joint Commission standards?"

Shapiro tugged on his already taught suspenders. "My client meets or exceeds all Joint Commission standards. Our latest report was exemplary."

Dan pounced. "Your client is out of compliance with MS 10.01.05 ep4, which states that hearing committees will include at least one peer, if investigating a clinical matter."

"My client has never been cited by The Joint Commission for a violation of this. If it pleases the court, I can provide the report from the last onsite survey."

Dan shook his head side to side. "Judge, Supreme Medical Center has agreed, as a condition of accreditation, to be in compliance with all Joint Commission standards at all times. The fact that a survey did not uncover this is immaterial."

Eat A Ton raised his voice. "Totally material! The Joint Commission has never cited us for that issue!"

"Your honor, hospital surveys are a sampling, if you will, of compliance, not a full 100% audit. If someone runs a stop sign, they have violated the law regardless of whether or not they received a ticket."

"Can you give me a copy of the Joint Commission standard?" The judge looked intrigued.

Dan was pleased to have gotten this far. He knew my goose was cooked if Eat A Ton was able to control the appeal the way he did the trial. "I have enclosed one in the brief packet, but I would be happy to give you another."

There was silence in the courtroom as Judge Robinson sifted through the packet until she found the document she wanted. She took another few minutes to carefully peruse the document. "Mr. Santucci, what are your exact requests?"

Dan spoke slowly but confidently. "We respectfully request that you require the appeal hearing to be scheduled before August 16th. We further respectfully request that the appeal be conducted in front a hearing panel. Finally, we request that the hearing panel include at least one peer, meaning a physician on active staff at Supreme Medical."

"Mr. Shapiro?"

Eat A Ton stood and looked flustered. His face was flushed. "First, there is no need to move up the appeal. The hospital requires the time to properly prepare our case. The hospital's duty to protect patients from substandard care far outweighs any inconvenience to the doctor involved. Second, there is no reason to change the appeal procedure since numerous Joint Commission inspections never cited this issue. Finally, your honor, Dr. Zander agreed to the use of the current procedure when he joined the staff."

Santucci was quick to object. "Your honor, the hospital held the first hearing less than ninety-six hours after the night of the incidents. They did that to be certain that my client was not totally prepared. And your honor, for that hearing my client was not permitted to retain counsel. Another example of how biased the by-laws are. In summary, when it suits the hospital, they can move quickly. When it suits their wishes to punish my client, they want to delay."

Shapiro countered. "Your honor, we follow the by-laws and rules and regulations. Time frames are not specified. We are free to schedule as we see fit. The first hearing was held as soon as possible to allow the medical staff to remove a dangerous physician from practicing further. Any delay in the hearing could have jeopardized patient's lives."

I jumped to my feet and glared at Eat A Ton. Dan and Azzie grabbed one arm each. I was ready to unleash a tirade of choice expletives when the sound of the rapping gavel brought back my senses. I sat down. I thought the gavel was rapping for me but Judge Robinson glared at the fat guy. "Mr. Shapiro I will tolerate no more theatrics. If I hear one more inciteful phrase such as dangerous physician or jeopardizing patient's lives, I WILL hold you in contempt. Do you understand me?"

Shapiro stood slowly with his head bowed. "Yes, your honor."

"Mr. Santucci please make a final response."

Dan looked over at me and then looked at the Judge. "Your honor, Mr. Shapiro has defamed my client by calling him dangerous. Thank you for your intervention. It should please the court to know that once Supreme Medical served my client with his notice of summary suspension he was suspended. Even if he was a "dangerous" physician he was not permitted to practice until the hearing was conducted. Since Supreme Medical elected to omit timeframes from their by-laws they were free to schedule the hearing when they had the information they needed. They chose to conduct it in a few days. Now they want six weeks for the appeal. We rest our case."

Judge Robinson again looked over her glasses. "I am recessing for lunch. Please return at 1:30 PM and I will issue my verdict. Court adjourned."

I waited until we had exited the courtroom and found our way to Mulligan's restaurant for lunch before asking. "Well, Dan what do you think?"

"Hard to tell. I found it encouraging that the judge took the time to read the Joint Commission standard. She could have dismissed its relevance out of hand. But I find it less encouraging that she elected to adjourn for lunch. As you can tell she doesn't fool around. If she was truly in agreement with us, I think we would have gotten an immediate verdict."

Azzie looked at Dan." Do you think that her anger at Shapiro will help us?"

"Very much so. He really pissed her off with that "dangerous doctor" comment."

I added. "That was clearly a mistake. I thought you said he was good?"

Dan quickly corrected me. "He is good, don't you ever forget that. But he was really taken aback when the judge read the Joint Commission standard. I watched him squirming in his seat. I am pretty sure that he thought he needed to underscore the magnitude of consequences here. He took a calculated risk that the judge would not know that a physician was suspended immediately when the charges were brought. He was hoping she would think that the lightning speed at which the hearing was held was for the benefit of the patients who might be subjected to a sub-par physician."

I was impressed. "You turned that right around on him and exposed the hypocrisy in the timing of the hearing and the appeal."

Dan rubbed his thumb to his index finger as if he was thumbing money. "That's what you pay the big bucks for, isn't it?"

We tried numerous talking points during lunch, but everything circled back to the upcoming ruling. If we lost, the farm and school were gone. If we won, we still had to win the appeal. It was an uphill battle.

At 1:20 we were back in our courtroom seats. Deuce just stared at me. One of those piercing stares. Since the judge hadn't appeared yet I used the opportunity to stick out my tongue at him. I was rewarded with a wicked kick by Azzie under the table.

"Ignore that asshole." She said loud enough for him to hear.

Just then Eat A Ton belched loudly as he pulled particles of lunch remnants off his massive chest and out of his beard. At precisely 1:30 the Judge appeared.

"Today, I am granting the injunction requested by Dr. Zander. It is the opinion of this court that a delay in the hearing beyond thirty days could irreparably harm Dr. Zander. In addition, the court notes that the hospital's objection to moving the appeal up is a stark contrast to the rapidity with which the hospital conducted the initial hearing. Therefore, I order for the appeal to occur on or before August 15th.

Furthermore, I am going to require that the appeal process utilizes a hearing panel to include at least one physician on the active staff of Supreme Medical. I am prepared to waive this requirement if the hospital can provide written documentation from The Joint Commission that their process as currently written does indeed meet Joint Commission standards. Any questions?"

Shapiro raised his hand. "Does the ruling preclude the use of a hearing officer to conduct the appeal, in addition to the use of a hearing panel?"

"Actually, in light of the rancor here, I find the use of a hearing officer to be an excellent idea. Provided the hearing officer's duties are to see that the appeal process conforms to the by-laws and that rules of law and decorum are followed. However, the hearing officer is to remain unbiased. The hearing officer is not to participate in any way in the deliberations and final decision of the hearing panel. Am I clear on this?"

Dan and Shapiro nodded and agreed.

"Court adjourned."

I was a good boy and stood there expressionless. Azzie let out a whoop that got a dirty look from Dan. Eat A Ton and Deuce looked pissed. Buster was shocked. It was clear that their team was not used to losing.

CHAPTER 38

Eat A Ton, Buster, and Deuce sat for a while in the courtroom reviewing the turn of events.

Shapiro started the discussion. "I didn't see this coming. Most judges won't get involved if you follow the bylaws, and we did."

Buster moaned. "I was worried about the hearing panel not including a physician. The physician surveyor from the Joint Commission questioned it during our survey last year."

Eat A Ton nodded. "That's right, you got me on a conference call and we talked him out of citing you. I remember that now."

Deuce mumbled. "So, I take it that is a moot point."

Eat A Ton nodded again. "We will never get it in writing from The Joint Commission that we are compliant because we clearly are not. We could file an appeal of this ruling, but I doubt we will prevail on the hearing panel or the date. We looked bad wanting to delay after having such a quick initial trial."

Deuce was ready to move on. "OK, next phase. Let's set the appeal date for Aug 16. Maybe someone will conveniently get sick that morning and we won't make the deadline. There are many ways that we can screw this kid."

Eat A Ton's head was about to come off from excessive shaking indicating no. "My guess is that if this appeal is not concluded by 3 PM Aug 15, Santucci will run right back to Judge Robinson."

Buster quipped. "So let him run."

Eat A Ton's voice increased in volume. "You two don't know this judge. She is not someone to lock horns with. If we do not complete the appeal in the time she gave us, she will move to dissolve all charges. Our best chance at winning this is to have the appeal done by 3 PM on the 15th. That doesn't mean we give up. After all, we still have a panel of three to be selected from the board members. We must include in that a physician from the board. The laypeople on the board will more than likely defer to the physician's judgment. So, if we choose a physician who shares our views, this will be over. Zander will be out, and he will not be able to own, train, or drive a harness horse until after his state hearing this fall. How many physicians are on the board, and who are they?"

Buster quickly responded. "Myself, Dr. Stanton, and Dr. Morehead."

Eat A Ton frowned. "Shit, that means we are stuck with Morehead."

Buster looked puzzled. "Why is that? Stanton and I are very familiar with the case. There is no question how either of us would vote."

"Bylaws, Dr. Hyman. They state that the board appeal committee must consist of three voting members of the board of directors. The judge has specified that one of those be a physician on the active staff. However, no one can be on the panel who was involved in the case or involved in the initial hearing. That takes you and Stanton out of the picture and puts Morehead in.

Deuce wasn't happy. "He is an odd duck. Smart, but very odd. Complains about little things and lets other bigger things go."

Buster agreed. "I can never read him. Sometimes he supports the medical staff leaders, and other times he throws darts. Hopefully I can talk some sense into him before the appeal."

Eat A Ton cautioned. "You will do nothing of the sort. Stay away from him. If he asks you about the case, tell him you can't talk about it. You can discuss the bylaws with him, and his responsibilities therewith, but nothing about the case."

Buster pleaded. "I can be discreet."

"Look, Dr. Hyman. If Morehead discloses that you spoke with him about the case Santucci would move to have him struck as a member of the committee. I would be powerless to oppose that. We have no other physicians to place on the panel and therefore we would likely forfeit. Case closed! Stay away from the board appeal members, and please tell the remainder of the medical executive committee to do the same."

They walked out of the courtroom and departed in their own vehicles. Deuce was not five feet out of the parking lot when he fired up his cell phone.

"Hello."

"Jenny, this is your Uncle Tom. Can I stop in for a minute?"

"Sure, Uncle Tom, would you like some dinner. I was going to order out."

"Maybe a drink, but no dinner. This won't take long."

1425 Jenny Rich's Apartment

Deuce sipped on a neat scotch as he summed up the day in court. Jenny was noticeably disturbed.

"I thought you told me that this was foolproof. Anyone with half of a brain will be able to see that he did no wrong and that he was framed. What the hell are we going to do now?"

"You, my niece, are going to calm down. Then you are going to plan how you wish to take care of this matter."

"Me? Me? Why me?"

"Because you have access to him. If you recall, I have evidence of a murder you committed in Florida that might find its way to the prosecutor's hands in Port Saint Lucie."

"How long are you going to hold that over my head?"

"OK, here's the deal. You take Zander out for good, and I will give you the evidence."

"What if you don't?"

"I will. I promise. See that he is gone before Millions Week. Thanks for the drink."

CHAPTER 39

Fired Up Farms
1430 July 25

Dan dropped Azzie and I off at the farm. He begged off a dinner invitation. He was already in attack mode. With less than three weeks to prepare, he had a ton of work to do. We planned to meet, or conference call daily, from now until the appeal.

I had already called Mom, and she had shared the good news with Stephanie. Stephanie greeted Azzie and me at the door. Stephanie's hair was messy, and her face was dirty, but she had a big smile on her face.

"I am so fucking happy I could just fart." She giggled and then ppppffffffttttttttttt! A loud and unmistakable anal emission of intestinal gases occurred.

"Excellent flavor too!" She proclaimed as she sniffed the air.

"Stephanie!" I screamed. But before I could get another word out, I got the Azzie eyes. That lady could give you a look that stopped you in your tracks and I just got one. I shut my mouth.

"It is great news isn't it, Stephanie? "Azzie changed the subject.

Mom walked out of the kitchen and joined the crowd. She sniffed and looked at Stephanie. "Again Stephanie? You got me about half sick in the car. What the hell did you eat?"

Stephanie tried to say something, but Mom interrupted her.

"Zachary, Azzie, that was really good news. I know we have a long way to go but at least we will get a chance. And before I forget, Joe called earlier."

I asked. "What did he say?"

"All he said was "Get the booze I've got some news.""

Azzie smiled "Knowing Joe, that could mean anything. Have a drink to celebrate good news or drink to drown out the thought of bad news."

Mom added, "he should be here around 4 pm, so we won't have long to wait."

Azzie turned to Stephanie. "Stephanie, do you want me to fix your hair?"

"Sure, are we going somewhere?"

"No, but I want to show you how to fix it better."

I added, "Right now it looks like you combed it with a dirty pitchfork."

That comment got me the Azzie eyes again. I decided to cut my losses.

"I am going over to the school for a sick call. I will be back before Joe gets here."

Mom returned to the kitchen as I wandered over to the school. Azzie and Stephanie climbed the stairs to the second-floor bathroom. Azzie made a pretense of washing her hands and offered Stephanie a washcloth to clean her face. Stephanie took it without question. Azzie led her to Azzie's room and had her sit in a chair facing a mirror.

"How about we comb your hair out, trim it a little, and give you a few curls?" Azzie asked.

Stephanie giggled and said, "Sure, make me fucking beautiful!"

Azzie set out to do just that. First, a lot of combing to get the tangles out. Then a trim followed by another trip to the bathroom to wash her hair. Azzie combed it out again and put in some curlers. She put Stephanie under the dryer and gave her a magazine to read. While her hair was drying Azzie went into her own closet and picked out some clothes that she thought would fit Stephanie. With about an eight-inch difference in their heights, that task proved to be difficult.

When Stephanie's hair was dry, Azzie carefully removed the curlers and went to work with a curling iron. Azzie used the opportunity to have a conversation.

"Stephanie, you have the potential to be quite a lady."

"Who in the hell cares about that?" Stephanie said as she continued to thumb through her magazine.

"As you get older you might get a little more interested in guys."

"I like guys, ZZ and his friends are great."

"No, I mean something more serious, like a boyfriend."

"Who in the hell would want me? I am goofed up in the head. I don't talk right, and I just don't see any guy getting interested in me."

"Farting hasn't helped you to attract men?" Azzie asked with a raised eyebrow.

Stephanie's face turned beet red. "I'm sorry."

"No need to be sorry Stephanie but in order to be treated like a lady you have to act like a lady."

"No fun in that."

"That's where you may be wrong. I have plenty of fun."

"But you are you! You are a big-shot celebrity, rich, beautiful, and brilliant. I am not."

"Well Stephanie, let me tell you something. You are what you make of yourself. And to this point in your life, you have done amazing things."

"Bullshit. I'm a fuck up."

Azzie spoke rapidly. "Oh really, how many, (she made air quotes as she spoke), fuck ups can make a life for themselves after being orphaned? How many fuck ups with forms of autism can gain independence? How many fuck up girls your age and size can handle a 1,000-pound animal like it was a small poodle being walked on a Sunday afternoon? How many? Not many. Stephanie, you are special, but you have been around guys too much."

"What's the matter with guys?"

"Nothing. They swear, they drink, they pass gas, and they think all of that is funny."

"It's not?"

"If you like being one of the boys it's ok, but if you want to be the girl that turns the boy's heads it's not."

The conversation continued after Stephanie's hair had been fixed. During a very painstaking application of makeup, and lipstick, Azzie went on to explain how guys think and what they like. Stephanie was all ears. She had never been exposed to a real lady. Most of the people at the track were men or boys or tomboys like her. Mom was sweet but she was also a tomboy. I was her best friend, but I was not a very good example of behaviors that a woman should emulate. Can you believe that?

Stephanie stared into the mirror. "Ok, I promise no more farting."

"So, you do see how that may turn some guys off?"

"Yeah, they might not want to go down on a girl who might cut one at any minute. It makes sense."

"Stephanie! We have a lot to discuss."

Stephanie eagerly put on the clothes Azzie had selected and turned to look again at herself in the mirror. What she saw made her cry. Long flowing curls of hair, beautifully manicured. Perfectly applied eye shadow and blush complimented her hair. Tastefully bright lipstick added the final touches to a stunning blue outfit that matched her eyes perfectly.

"What do you think Stephanie?"

"I can't fffff," she stopped before the f bomb exploded, then she started again. "I can't believe that is me. I am gorgeous." Tears ran down her cheeks.

"Yes, you are sweetheart, now quit crying before you fucking ruin my makeup job."

"See, you swear too!!!"

"And guess what Stephanie? I even pass gas on occasion. But don't tell anyone. I blame it on the dog. Being a lady involves a lot of secrets."

They both laughed.

"Azzie, how long have you had a thing for Joe?"

Azzie was visibly shaken by the question. "Joe is great, but we are just friends."

Stephanie quickly countered. "BS, you and ZZ are friends. You act different around Joe."

Azzie thought for a moment. "Now you are imagining stuff. Maybe the hairspray got you high."

"Oh really, I see how you look at him. I see that when he is around you, stand taller and straighter and that your boobs stick out more. You always look nice but when he is around you look nicer."

Azzie had no idea what to say. She started to mumble something. Stephanie had struck a nerve. Fortunately, her thoughts were interrupted by the unmistakable sound of Joe coming in the front door.

CHAPTER 40

Fired Up Farms
1630 July 25

"Boom, Boom, Boom. The king is here and I need a beer." Bellowed Joe as he crossed the threshold. I was right behind him having finished my business at the school.

I pounded my chest with my right arm and said, "So it is written, so it shall be done." I always thought I would have made a cool Roman emperor. I went to the kitchen to get the drinks as I shouted to the group at the door, "Go to the living room we will debrief there."

Mom greeted Joe as I delivered the beverages. I had a beer for Joe and a Snapple for myself. Joe was about to object to my choice of drink when it hit him.

"Driving tonight?"

"Yep, three races starting with the fourth. Save me a beer for when I get home."

There was a knock on the door. I jumped to answer it and found PC standing on the front porch.

"What are you doing here?" I asked.

"Great to see you too, ZZ." PC looked hurt.

"Sorry, I knew you were off tonight, and I didn't expect you. Please come in."

"No problem bro. Actually, that Saunders kid got sick and I am collecting piss tonight. I want to get your input before I go to work."

"Input or sure tips on what to bet?"

"Same thing." PC had his program in his back pocket.

Joe overheard the conversation and wandered to the door. I introduced him to PC. "Joe Crinelli, please meet Johnson Stevens, a good friend. He goes by PC."

Joe lurched forward and gave PC a bear hug. "A good friend of ZZ's is a friend of mine for life." He continued. "How do you get PC out of Johnson Stevens? ZZ, you have a way with nicknames."

PC explained how he collects equine urine samples at the racetrack using a cup on a stick. Hence his moniker, "Pisscatcher."

Joe remembered that Azzie had added him to one of the teams, but he did not know the significance of the name until now. He cut loose a belly laugh and emptied his beer. "I need another beer, PC can I get you one?"

PC declined the beer but agreed to a black coffee. Mom told Joe to stay put and went to the kitchen to fill the drink orders.

PC opened the program on the coffee table as we all sat down to review the evening's races. Our attention was quickly diverted.

Azzie slowly came down the steps. I noticed for the first time how Joe's eyes followed her every movement.

"Sweet cheeks, my are you beautiful." Joe proclaimed. I sensed no jokes or smart responses in his remarks. Joe was sincere and that was unusual. Azzie looked flustered by the compliment. Azzie never looked flustered. I was trying to process the contradictions when my brain flashed tilt in vivid vibrating colors.

Down the steps behind Azzie came a blonde bombshell. The only word that came to my dizzy mind was "hottie." Stephanie was not wearing a ball cap, jeans, or dirty clothes. She was a babe, and I was shocked.

PC ran to the steps and extended his hand. Stephanie took it and he helped her walk gracefully off the landing. I had never seen her do anything graceful when she was not piloting a horse around the track. She looked at Azzie and smiled. Then she stood straighter and thrust her chest out. WTF was going on? Stephanie walked PC over to Azzie and introduced her. Where did those manners come from?

I had no idea what the hell was happening but I didn't have the time to find out just yet. I had to leave in forty-five minutes for the track. I spoke up. "Can we get to the living room to debrief?"

PC said, "I can leave if you want privacy."

I replied, "PC, you are one of the family, you are welcome to stay until you need to leave for the track."

Stephanie spoke. "Please PC, stay for a few minutes." She somehow found a chair beside his.

PC agreed. One look at him and I knew he was smitten. He and I had been friends for many years both on and off the track. I never knew him to be interested in anything except betting on races and fantasy football. My head was on fire. Too much information to process in a short period of time.

Mom brought me back to earth.

"ZZ, please give us the details on the hearing?"

In light of the time constraints, I gave the abbreviated version.

"Dan is a damn wizard. We got a ruling that the appeal must be done on or before 8/15. AND," I emphasized the AND, "they have to use at least one physician on their panel."

Joe took another swig of beer. "Sounds like case closed to me."

"Sorry Joe, we still have a long way to go. There will be at least one physician on the panel, and we have to convince a panel of three. We figure any lay people will follow the physician's lead, so convincing the physician is paramount. Knowing how inbred their medical staff is, the road is uphill."

Joe nodded. "Agreed, but at least there is some hope. Speaking of hope, I was hoping that Dan would still be here. Can we get him on the phone?"

Mom got Dan on the line and placed him on the speakerphone. I started the conversation.

"Dan, can you hear us?"

"Got you, go ahead."

"Joe has some news that he wanted you to hear," I said as I took my seat.

Joe quickly took his cue. "I hope you are sitting counselor." He paused but before Dan could answer Joe blurted, "I think Carl will be joining us soon."

The room erupted in cheers. Joe gave a brief synopsis of his findings. He added that the state police detective that he shared the video with would not commit to a new trial but Joe was very, very, hopeful.

Azzie jumped up and kissed Joe on the mouth. Stephanie screamed and PC just stared at her with his mouth open. The way this was going we were going to need more rooms.

Dan, of course, wanted copious details that Joe was more than willing to provide. I voiced that I had to get to the track along with PC, Mom, and Stephanie. We decided to have a team meeting on Sunday afternoon at the farm. Dan asked Joe to call him back in thirty minutes and hung up.

PC stood and looked at me. "Ok ZZ, how do you feel?"

"Great," I said.

"That's disappointing," PC replied.

Everyone in the room stared at PC.

Then without thinking, I said, "I don't give a shit."

"That's better!" PC said with a grin.

Joe asked, "What's the difference?"

PC explained. "I have watched ZZ drive his entire career. At his best, when he doesn't give a shit, he dominates a race with his confidence. He's like the Starship Enterprise, he goes where no one has gone before. After his accident the best he was, was good. When he is good, he wins most races he is supposed to win, the ones where he has the best horse. When he doesn't give a rip, he does amazing things on the track that mere mortals cannot do. He wins with many horses that should not have won. He picks them up and carries them over the wire. This summer he has been good. I know he can be better."

Joe asked me "Are you sure ZZ?"

"Yep, with your news on Carl and my win in court, I am getting fired up. When I get fired up there is no race I cannot win."

PC concluded, "Case closed."

I gathered my things for the track. I had to interrupt PC making chit-chat with Stephanie. "C'mon PC get a move on. I'm in the third race and I don't need another fine for missing the breathalyzer deadline."

Stephanie ran back up the steps to change. Before I could get PC out the door Azzie called everyone except Stephanie into the kitchen.

"Can I get a little help here?" Azzie sounded irritated.

Joe ran to her side, but she brushed him off.

"I need help from all of you, ZZ, PC, Joe, Mom, all of you. When we get the whole group together, I need their help too."

Joe nodded. "Name it, sweet cheeks, anything you want."

Azzie spoke slowly. "I want all of you to stop treating Stephanie as one of the boys. She is quite a young lady, but she thinks she needs to act like all of you to impress you."

I protested. "C'mon Azzie, she IS one of us."

Azzie rebuked me. "I can't believe someone as smart as you can be so stupid at times." She turned to face PC. "PC, I saw you drooling when she came down the steps."

PC was obviously embarrassed. "You did? I ah, I ah, Ok, so you did. She looked so great. I never saw her look like that. I couldn't help but stare."

Azzie acknowledged the admission. "Bingo. Now look, I know you all love her dearly and you want nothing but the best for her. You all adopted her, and she became one of the boys. Excuse me, but I think you know what I mean. Anyway, I can show her how to dress, and groom, and apply makeup but only you folks can encourage her to act more like a lady."

Joe laughed. "Shit, we have to show her how to be bitchy when she has PMS?"

Azzie just gave Joe the eyes and he slumped into a kitchen chair, duly chastised.

Azzie continued. "I mean the language, the farting, belching, scratching, and all the manly things you do. Those actions might in a sick way make each of you more charming, but they make Stephanie anything but."

I stared at the floor. That really hit home. I had been one of the biggest influences on Stephanie's life. I laughed when it happened, but I was really embarrassed when she passed gas today. I never wanted to be embarrassed by Stephanie. No one spoke for a minute, then I got the courage to address Azzie.

"Azzie, point taken. The woman I saw come down those steps today deserves our support. She is incredibly special, and I for one, have done little to help her be the best she can be. Thank you for assisting her. I will change."

Mom was crying. Azzie put her arm around her. "Mom don't blame yourself; you also have been surrounded by too much testosterone. It takes me a few days after hanging out with Joe to clean up my language. We don't need to do anything drastic, but can we all tone it down a little?"

Joe's normal response would have been a smart-ass comment Tonight, it was "you bet."

All things in due time.

PC and I ran out the door. Mom and Stephanie would come along separately. Joe and Azzie decided to stay and watch the races from home. I had my doubts that they would see any of the races. Good for them. I did ask them to set up a team meeting for Sunday afternoon August 3. Joe would inform Dan when he called him back. PC or I would get word to Father Jonathan.

CHAPTER 41

Miracle Mile Racetrack and Casino
1755 July 25

I originally had five drives tonight. Two from our barn and three catch drives. When I was suspended two of the catch drives disappeared. But one trainer elected to leave me up in the hope I would drive. I owe him a big "thank you."

At least all three horses looked competitive. Taco was the favorite to win her race. Rio was about 5:1 morning line odds. As usual, Supreme Stables had a horse in a bunch of races, but Billie was not on the bike for them. WTF? He had been replaced for tonight by Nick Demary. He was known as "The Blue Man" as his colors were very blue. Although he wasn't the top driver, he had quite a following at the track.

After warming up a few horses I got a coffee and sat down in the driver's room. Blue Man was holding court with a number of drivers who liked to listen to his stories. I wasn't sure if they were listening to him, or laughing at him, but they made quite a racket. I took my program and headed to the paddock. Where the hell was Billie? He wasn't driving at all. Was he sick?

A few minutes later I was walking down the aisle in the paddock while looking at my program. I ran right into a mountain of a man. He shoved me.

"Watch where you are going, asshole." Little John said angrily.

"Yo, Lurch, you better stay out of my way, or I'll kick your ass," I said looking up at the giant.

Little John mumbled as he walked away. When he got to his horse's stall, he opened the note I had slid in his pocket. "Team meeting

1400 this Sunday at the farm. Lunch at 1200. Make sure you are not followed."

I got a kick out of the cloak-and-dagger stuff. But on a serious note, we all knew that if Deuce or any of the Supremes figured out that Little John was Father Jonathan he could be in danger. So, we passed notes on occasion. He also had a supply of burner phones that he kept somewhere in the woods near the groom's quarters. He was certain that they searched his truck and room frequently. He never used his cell phone or computer to contact us.

One of the grooms filled me in on Billie. Supposedly they fired him and replaced him with Blue Man. No one was sure exactly why. There were rumors that Deuce was still pissed about us claiming Supreme Taco and turning her around. Why that got blamed on Billie and not the trainer baffled me. But the final straw in Billie's coffin was his kneeling in front of Stephanie. Wow, Billie got taken out in the war against us. It was obvious, and this just confirmed it, that we, (my family, our stable, and the school), were the targets here. Why?

Mom arrived in the paddock right on time with Taco. Mom was an interesting character. Worked hard from daylight to sunset and never complained. Did what she could to maintain a family, a marriage, a racing operation, and a school. She was the quietest one in the family. She didn't speak often but when she did you had better listen. She was incredibly wise and a superb judge of character.

She had the biggest grin on her face, and she was humming one of her favorite church hymns when she walked by with Taco. She often hummed when she worked, especially when she was happy. Tonight, I knew why she was happy. Her and Carl were not overly affectionate. I had heard that their marriage had some rough times, mostly when my dad was tanked. But she endured and persevered. Tonight, she looked exceptionally beautiful. That Azzie must be gussyying up the entire house!

In just a few minutes Mom had Taco ready to warm up. I looked her over and double-checked the equipment. Satisfied, I walked beside Mom as we walked to the entrance to the track.

"Pretty exciting day, Mom. I was thrilled that Dan got us some justice and of course, I am so happy about Carl." Before she could comment I continued. "I am sorry that I was so quick to believe that he was guilty. I really should have pushed harder for an investigation."

"Water under the bridge Zachary, but you can help him get rid of some of his guilt."

"Dan will take care of that."

"That's not what I mean. Your father was hurt more by the rift that developed between you two than going to prison. Of course, he felt very guilty when he thought he had killed Ken, but his loss of your respect was more than he could bear."

"Oh." I wanted to say more but my brain and mouth had frozen in thought.

I grabbed the lines and jumped on Taco's sulkey. She had really come a long way. She had been a dismal performer for Supreme Stables. With a little TLC, she had turned into quite a racehorse for Fired Up Farms. As we entered the track, I thought back to the night that she broke her maiden. PC and Jenny had watched in the clubhouse and joined us in the winner's circle. Mr. G inquired about Jenny. He missed her.

"Mr. G, you know that Dan was emphatic that I have no contact with her until after the trial. And If I don't have any contact, you are shit out of luck. Go back to sleep." Yes, all men have names for, and talk to their dicks.

I jogged slowly on the first lap and got the usual hellos and f.u.'s from the racing fans camped at the rail. That stuff used to bother me, but with what I have been through lately, I was able to tune them out. As we continued up the rail toward the ¾ pole I heard a familiar sound, screaming kids.

At the top of the stretch was tonight's edition the Autistic Army. Thirty special kids with thirty special teachers. Usually, we only brought fifteen kids, but Stephanie insisted on all of them coming to see Rio. All sixty were screaming and jumping up and down as Taco approached. I slowed Taco down and stopped her in front of the crowd. I pulled gently on the left line and Taco knelt down on her left knee, bowing to the crowd. They went nuts. I pulled Taco back up and we continued our warmup laps.

"How is she?" Mom asked as we walked back into the paddock.

"About half lame."

"Do you want to scratch her?"

"No, let's see how she is next warmup. I'll probably just race her easy."

Mom went to work removing equipment so she could give Taco a nice hot bath. I tried hard not to smile. That horse was as sound as could be, and we both knew it. She almost ran off with me at the end of the warmup. But there were ears everywhere at the racetrack. Most of them were pointed at the horses in each race with a chance to win. Everyone was looking for an inside tip. Nothing like a little disinformation to muddy the waters.

I got over to the paddock that contained Chantilly Lace. Her trainer was Desmond Wallace. He was stabled at The Meadows, but he had shipped Chantilly out to compete in some NJ sire stakes races. She was eligible because she had been bred in NJ. Billy had been driving her for the past two starts here in Jersey. She had a third and a win. Tonight, was the $150,000 final in the three-leg series and she was 3/1. I had never met the man, but he called me this week and asked me to drive Chantilly. I had seen his picture and recognized him immediately. I offered my hand.

"Mr. Wallace, thank you for the opportunity. I really appreciate your support by sticking with me during the suspension. It's my pleasure to finally meet you."

"ZZ, thank you for taking over. I was shocked when Billie had to jump off these drives. This filly is just coming into her own and you know how he likes to showboat big races."

"Yeah," I laughed, "With Billy, the show is sometimes better than the race. What happened?"

"I heard he had an exclusive with Supreme Stables and his contract even had a noncompete. They weren't enforcing it when he was originally driving for me, but something changed. He can't drive at any track on any night that they have a horse in for six months."

I blurted out, "Wow, what kind of asshole would sign a contract like that?"

Before he could answer I said, "Billie would. Billie would have seen the flash of cash and signed."

Mr. Wallace shook his head in agreement.

I ended a short but uncomfortable silence. "Now how did you pick me? Don't get me wrong, I really, really, need the drive and I am grateful that you chose me."

"I watched this kid come up through the ranks a few years ago. He made all the right moves at all the right times. He beat many of my horses with his head and his hands. My horses had more ability, but he had more talent than my drivers. I was about to ask him to drive some for me when my horse took a bad step and stepped on his face."

"That was your horse?"

"Sorry, it was. I was hoping to make it up to you."

"Consider it made up." We shook hands. "Now tell me about Chantilly."

The story was straightforward. She had some speed but wasn't a speed demon. She was decent gaited but she sometimes broke if she got uptight or pushed too hard. Although she didn't have a ton of speed off the gate she raced better near the front. All of that was trainer speak for "don't count your commission check just yet, and don't plan on a big one."

I changed my mind after I warmed her up. She seemed sharp to me. And since I am in my "I don't give a shit stage" I just might roll her out of the gate. I didn't tell Mr. Wallace. He seemed like the kind of trainer that really didn't want to know. He put a driver up for a reason and he let the driver succeed or cook his own goose. My kind of trainer.

I handed the lines back to Mr. Wallace just as Stephanie entered the paddock with Rio. Rio was a superbly built filly and she was decked out perfectly. White lines and equipment to match my colors. Stephanie was also decked out. Sure, she had on jeans, but they were clean and more tight fitting than usual. They were complimented by a white button-down shirt that was tied tightly under her bosoms. She never looked that good at the track. All eyes in the paddock were on her.

"Got milk?" I said as I eyed her suddenly prominent breasts.

She blushed and was about to unleash a tirade of vulgarity when she just laughed.

PC was wandering around, getting his gear together to catch the horse piddle. He just stared at Stephanie.

"PC, you better reel that tongue of yours back in before a horse steps on it," I chided.

"ZZ, sorry I just can't believe how beautiful she is. It was always there; I just never saw it."

My witty retort was interrupted when the paddock judge called. One of the drivers was late. Would I drive Little Sniffer in the third race?

CHAPTER 42

Miracle Mile Racetrack and Casino

2000 July 25

Little Sniffer seemed live as I scored her down. Nick was driving Badlands for Supreme Stables. He was favored and my horse was the second favorite. Now getting under Nick's skin was different than getting Billie fired up. Billie was easy. I just stuttered and made fun of him like mean kids did in school. I hated doing it because of the struggles I saw our kids put up with. But when Supreme Stables was hell-bent on ruining us there was no mercy to be shown.

Nick was a blabbermouth and a control freak. I knew if I could shut him up and put doubts in his head, I may have a chance. As we were warming up down the backside, we found our horses in close proximity. He just glared at me, and I smiled back.

"Congratulations Blue Balls, now you are driving for the devil." I hoped that Nick liked his new name.

"Hey ZZ, your sister is smoking hot tonight. Too bad your horses aren't."

Nick and I were side by side as we approached the starting gate. A few seconds before the start I said "Nick, is your tire going flat?"

He looked down as the gate opened. It was just enough of a delay on his part that I got Little Sniffer to the front easily. I heard a horse coming up on the outside of me as we neared the ¼ mile pole. I knew it was Nick and that he wanted to get the top and then slam on the breaks.

I shook the lines and Sniffer took the hint. We sped up and we parked Nick's horse out. He tried the whole way down the stretch to get by and Sniffer and I managed to keep the lead. Now I could see him seething. I was in the prick's head and now was the time to add insult to injury.

"Hey Nick, how do you like it out there?"

"Fuck you, Zander, you will pay big for this."

"Adios asshole," I screamed. I gave Blue Man the famous Zander salute and let Little Sniffer drive on. Badlands faded badly at the ¾ pole and Sniffer won by five lengths.

Ten minutes later Mom just smiled and hummed as we walked Taco out to the track.

"You got the Blue Man singing the blues."

"You haven't heard him even begin to sing Mom!" I promised.

Nick stayed away from me in the warmup, and we were as far apart as we could get at the gate. He had the rail with Supreme Showboat, and I had the nine-hole. Taco was super handy. I could leave for position or duck her. But with the nine-hole, ducking wasn't such a great option. It was very difficult to come from dead last and win. She had done it but against less competition. Tonight, she was in the Filly and Mare Open pace. That was a race for the best female pacers on the grounds. Almost every horse had the ability to leave. I had to be careful. But how can you be careful if you don't give a ....?

I looked down the line and saw that about half of the drivers were itching to get to the front. I decided to roll out of the gate and then see what I could work out. We got out of there flying but we were not able to get to the pylons. Supreme Showboat was in the lead. The five horse was first over on the outside and we were behind the five. As a spot opened up at the pylons, I attempted to back Taco into it but Sam Goodwin pulled the five down and into the spot. That left me sitting on the outside. I could see Blue Balls pulling back on the reins. He figured he had the front locked up and he wanted to save his horse. I was six lengths back and he obviously didn't think I was coming to the top.

Score no points for that guess BB. I downshifted Taco into another gear. She flew up on the outside and grabbed the lead. By the time BB started his horse up I was past him. He immediately pulled back to the outside and retook the lead. I did not want to park him out. I could have done it but that would necessitate giving up any chance of winning the race. Although I wanted to ruin the Supremes and Blue Balls, my main job was to win the race.

BB slowed down the third quarter as he usually did. I had watched his horse race her last three starts and I knew that her weak spot was the last 1/8 mile. Her last quarters were twenty-eight seconds at best and last 1/16 was usually around fifteen seconds. As expected, BB knew that well and when he hit the ¾ pole he let her loose to run away from the pack. He was hoping to get a big enough lead that she could hang on. That was the smart play. He opened a two-length lead when I set Taco down for the stretch drive. I expected to close in quickly. In fact, I was more worried about the horses behind me than I was about Showboat.

That was an errant thought. Showboat flew down the stretch and won easily. I was so flummoxed that she got away from me that I almost let Taco get beat for a second. Luckily for me, she knew what needed to be done and did it without me. Now my head was the one that had been invaded. How in the hell did that horse, (Showboat), throw in that last quarter? She went in 26:4. I would have to watch the tape to see how she did the last 16th but it was much faster than she ever had done before. All I could think was "Better living through biochemistry." WTF did Supremes give that horse this week?

I had little time to ponder that dilemma as Chantilly was in the next race. Chantilly Lace turned out to be a dream. I had wanted to try to get the top with her out of the gate, but she got away fifth. I pulled her out at the half and sent her after the leader. Our dear friend Blue Balls had the lead. As we pulled up beside him, he screamed over.

"How do YOU like it out there?"

"Just loving it asshole. Kiss my grits." I followed that witty repartee up with a Zander salute. I shook the lines, and the filly kicked it in gear. We opened a 3 ½ length lead that held up in the stretch. Chantilly banked $75,000 and I got $3,750. Pretty nice score. Plus, she was very live for an even bigger race during Millions Week. I was singing as I waltzed over to Rio's stall. It was one of my favorite songs.

"My girl can't wrestle but you ought to see her box."

Stephanie shook her head and said, "How juvenile."

"Stephanie, you of the new do (referring to her recent coiffing by Azzie), are you going to become a stick in the mud now?"

"Eat shit ZZ"

"That's my girl!"

"Rio is keyed up. Get her away from the field in the post-parade and try to get her onto the grass. She likes that."

"Ok, anything else?"

"Yeah, when you drop the hammer, don't fall off the bike." She let out a huge belly laugh.

Rio was keyed up. I did as Stephanie directed. As she walked slowly through the infield grass, she did settle. But, of course, who came charging up next to us but Blue Balls and Supreme Dream. It startled the recently calmed Rio, who freaked out. She reared and nearly ended up in my lap. Luckily, she came back down on her front feet and we took off. I hit something in the infield and flattened one of my tires. I informed the outrider who notified the starter. There was a race delay as I went back to get a new race bike.

Stephanie was fit to be tied. Her newly sanitized vocabulary was trashed for a tirade that was amazing even for her. I got the bike hooked up and headed back to the track. I needed to get this horse to the starting gate soon. She was wound up and was about to get washed out and done.

As the starter pulled the car away, I realized that there was no point in trying to get her off the gait. I was surprised she didn't jump over it. But the good news was that once she got to the top, she let me get a hold of her. She seemed to be trotting within herself. So, I thought. The quarter was in 27.3. I almost shit. Way too fast. I was hoping for 28.3 or even 29 seconds. Now BB's horse was banging her chin on my helmet.

I knew if I backed Rio down that he would pull. So, I let her motor on. Half in 56.3 seconds. Way too fast for a green horse. I really hated to gut her this early in her career.

BB pulled down the back side and we raced side by side. Funny thing though. Rio was still going strong but she acted relaxed. It was like Rocky taking hits to his head and toying with Apollo Creed. She was racing and she was liking it a lot. Third quarter was 1:25.4. The announcer was going bonkers. As we rounded the final turn, there they were. The Awesome Army. Tonight, they were all there. They had watched this horse train for months and she acted like a pet around them. I saw them all jumping up and down. I mean all of them, kids and therapists. They were waving their left arms up and down like they were hammering a board.

That meant only one thing to me and Rio. They wanted us to put the hammer down and end the race. Well, who was I to deny thirty special kids? I cut her loose and she responded with amazing speed and grace. She finished strong and clocked her mile in 1:54.2. Unheard of time for only her third start. She wasn't even breathing all that hard when I pulled her up.

It was sheer bedlam in the winner's circle. The poor photographer had a hell of a time getting a picture. Getting thirty special needs kids to do anything together was a big task. But finally, she got it done and we went back to the paddock. PC waved his magic cup and Rio pissed up a storm. That would help us get home sooner.

I would have been done but the judges conned me into a drive in the last race. The driver who was late never made it. At least the last drive was exciting. A little too exciting for me. Crock Pot was a puller, and he about pulled my arms out of their sockets to keep him under control. By the half-mile pole, I was tired and he was really going at it. I laid back in the bike and pulled for all I could when Crock Pot collapsed on the track. I was thrown in the air and landed on the track on my left side. I heard screams and hoofs. I pulled myself into a ball and waited to get stepped on again.

When the expected death did not come, I opened my eyes. I saw Crock Pot lying on the track. Suddenly he woke up and tried to stand. I jumped up and knelt on his neck to keep him down until I got help. Luckily, help arrived. We got the equipment off Crock Pot and stood him up. He didn't look any worse for wear. He had "choked down." He was pulling hard, and that made me tug as hard as I could on the reins. His air got cut off. He blacked out. Suddenly I realized that I too felt ok. You see when I don't give a shit it all works out.

CHAPTER 43

Fired Up Farms
1000 August 3

Father Jonathan arrived at 10 AM. He knew that the meeting was at 2 PM but he thought some people may want to attend mass. He had said that he wasn't a priest when he arrived, but he might have to confess that he lied. He was a true priest, and he couldn't wait to say mass for his friends. Plus, he did not want to miss Sunday lunch. Mom put out a tremendous spread. Living at the track for a few weeks made him miss good cuisine

"Padre, were you followed?"

"No, my son," laughed Father Jonathan.

"Good deal." I said as I hugged him.

"Father, can I get you some breakfast?" Mom ran out and kissed him.

"Raincheck on breakfast but you got me for lunch."

What started out as a small mass in the living room of our house turned into a great tribute to God held at the school. In a little over an hour, an altar was set up and chairs were arranged. Many of the kids and their handlers arrived. They were Catholics or their parents had specified that they had no issue with religious teachings. No children were required to attend.

Mom, Stephanie, PC, and all of the "Dying Was Easy" group were there. Somehow Azzie ended up sitting next to Joe and PC ended up right beside Stephanie. Stephanie had on a beautiful yellow sundress that I had never seen before. I was sure that Azzie took her shopping.

Father Jonathan said an amazing mass. His sermon was focused on how right will outperform wrong every time. He sat in front of the children as he mesmerized them with his words. I was amazed how such a big man could get so "small" to speak face-to-face with the kids. His words were carefully chosen to reach kids who were hard to reach. He was an incredible person.

Dan arrived at 1 PM. Right on time for a great dinner. Mom, Azzie, and Stephanie had outdone themselves. I was shocked that Stephanie had participated. Prior to today, I thought Stephanie only knew that the kitchen was a room on the way to the barn. She wanted to learn how to cook. Wow.

Dinner, after a tremendous salad selection, consisted of a very tender pork roast, mashed potatoes, and home-grown green beans with onions. The dessert was homemade apple pie with vanilla ice cream. After coffees all around the group adjourned to the library.

I opened the meeting. "On behalf of my family and the Always Hope School, I can't thank each and every one of you enough. Your work to this point, and your help going forward, is a gift from God. Ok, let's get to it. Let's start with Joe."

"Thanks ZZ. Boom, boom, boom. We have in our possession, and more importantly, the state police, have a superb video that shows conclusive evidence that Carl Zander was not driving the truck that killed Ken Harrow."

He waited for effect even though everyone already knew that news.

"I can add that I have shared this with the district attorney and she is supportive of our cause."

I clapped my hands and asked. "When can Carl get out of jail?"

"When the district attorney agrees to a new trial we can proceed." Dan answered.

I pressed Dan. "Isn't there any other way? We need Carl here."

Dan quipped. "Dah, if the governor would get involved maybe. But that's not realistic."

I calmly said, "Hold on."

I dialed my phone as they all watched.

"Governor? Sorry to bother you, ZZ Zander here. Do you mind if I put you on speakerphone?"

The governor questioned whether I was amongst friends. As an experienced politician, he was leery of being on a speakerphone.

I reassured him and he agreed to others hearing the conversation.

"Oh ZZ, good to hear from you, how can I help?" he inquired.

I explained briefly to the governor about Carl. Then Dan filled him in about the case. When Dan finished that subject, he asked the governor if he could intervene in my license suspension. The governor patiently got the details of that issue and promised he would call us back in an hour.

At the conclusion of the call, Dan shook his head and asked, "How in the hell do you know the governor?"

"His son had an infection that the governor did not want to become public knowledge."

Azzie was incredulous. "So, he picks your name out of a phone book and asks you to take care of it?"

There was copious laughter from the group.

"No smart ass. Before we all hooked up in college I volunteered for his campaign. At that time, he was running for state senator."

Joe jumped in "He remembered you from way back then?"

I was losing my patience. "If everyone would hold the questions, I will be happy to explain."

I was glad to hear silence. "I was racing and making pretty good money when he first ran for governor. I contributed heavily to his campaign and met him at a fundraiser at the track."

Father Jonathan couldn't resist the temptation. "I can hear the conversation now. 'ZZ thank you for your support. I hope I can count on you if my son ever gets gonorrhea.'"

My face got red but then I quickly joined in the very loud laughter. "Ok here's how it went down. I was working outside of Atlantic City. While on duty I got a call from a representative of the governor. It took about ten minutes for me to get the gist of the cryptic request he was making. The governor's staff was concerned about any negative publicity now for the governor, or later for the young man. They had called every ER within a fifty-mile radius of his son's dorm inquiring as to the name of the ER doctor on duty. They first checked the licensing board to find out about any sanctions and then they checked their donor lists. Once they saw how supportive I had been of the governor they made the call. And, who said he had gonorrhea? Public record or not, I do have a duty of confidentiality to him. So, to be clear, I never specified what type of infection."

Dan was quick to reply. "Fair enough, but medical records ARE confidential, by law. That whole business seemed like overkill."

"So are sealed court proceedings, but they just so happen to become public during certain elections. Didn't Barack Obama win some election in Illinois after a "sealed" divorce proceeding record of an opponent suddenly became unsealed?"

Dan was speechless.

"The governor didn't want his son to be harmed in the future if it leaked. So, I treated him. I made a record of my treatment in case the state board ever came snooping around. I have it in my personal file. It just isn't a hospital record that political opponents might be able to reach."

"Oh, aren't we the clever one." Dan laughed and the room erupted in applause and laughter.

When the noise dissipated Father Jonathan went next. He was clearly exasperated. He knew the Supremes were as dirty as could be, but he had absolutely no proof. The horses he groomed were winning often but other than race day half of them were dead lame. They almost never trained and when they did, it was light. He questioned how were they so good on race day? His conclusion was PEDS, (performance enhancing drugs). He bolstered his deduction with some data. A surprising number of the horses that the Supremes claimed won their first start. It was a far higher percentage of first-start wins than any other trainer had at the track. Whatever they were using, it had to be something that worked quickly. Something like a milkshake or a tranquilizer.

He went on to report that he knew that many of the things used to dope horses had been invented and perfected by Olympic contestants. That's why he stopped watching the Olympics. He was sure that many athletes were clean, but when it came to light years ago that many top Olympic swimmers were "milkshaking," he never watched again.

They were drinking large amounts of bicarbonate in various forms prior to competition. When an athlete, or any person or horse, exercises they build up lactic acid in their system. The lactic acid makes them tired and decreases performance. The bicarbonate buffers the acid, and, boom, boom, boom, improved performance.

Unscrupulous trainers had perfected a way to do it with horses. Damn animals wouldn't drink the horrid stuff but that was solved with the insertion of a nasogastric tube. Very easy to insert into a horse. Once in, they poured their concoction in there a few hours prior to the race and cashed many winning tickets a couple hours later. Not to mention the hefty purse winnings check that came 7-10 days later.

"I have no solid evidence. I am sure they are drugging their horses something awful, but I haven't seen it. I haven't found any drugs or needles in the barn. No one that I was able to confidentially talk to had seen anything of significance." Father Jonathan ended his remarks.

I added, "Couple that with negative post-race drug tests and they look clean."

Father Jonathan muttered. "I would swear they are not. Plus, can anyone here explain this quiet time crap?"

Azzie spoke up "Quiet time?"

I stood to make sure everyone could hear me. "Yeah, these whackos close up their barn at 1 PM on race day. No one is permitted in or out until 3 PM other than the trainer and the head of security for Supreme Stables. They claim to play calming music and soothe the horses."

Father Jonathan added "That's right. That could easily be the time that they do their dirty work. None of the grooms are allowed in during that time. But again, we have nothing but suspicions."

Joe interrupted. "Can they lock a barn? Aren't there fire regulations?"

Father Jonathan quickly answered. "Yes, but they installed an automatic fire suppression system. With that in place, they are free to lock up."

CHAPTER 44

Fired Up Farms
1530 August 3

My phone rang. "Hello, governor."

He was nervous about any further speakerphone performances, so I kept the conversation private. The group could still hear my end. "Sure, we can get someone up there tomorrow. 9 AM, no problem. We will be there. I can't thank you enough." I just listened for the next few minutes before responding to the governor.

"Governor, I totally understand. With the controversy that the Dagostino case created, I can see how you have to keep your distance. Thank you for the help with Carl. Can I ask one small additional favor?"

Before I hung up, I asked the Governor to see what he could do to make Deputy Taser more responsive to the needs of the public. He laughed and said he would make a few calls later. Deputy Taser would never know why his career went into the toilet. He deserved it.

After I hung up, I was happy to fill in the blanks for the group.

The governor commuted Carl's sentence. He also spoke with the attorney general who will personally manage the paperwork to give Carl a new trial to expunge his record. He could have pardoned him, but he didn't want any political ramifications. The attorney general assured the governor that with the evidence the police currently had in their possession, Carl would ultimately be cleared. But he was free to come home tomorrow morning.

All hell broke loose. There was screaming, crying, hooting, and hollering. Tears of joy covered most cheeks. Joe was hugging Azzie and somehow Stephanie ended up in PC's arms. I twirled Mom around like a rag doll. Dan and Father Jonathan were dancing. It was just plain nuts.

Dan piped up as the crowd calmed a little. "Do you want me to arrange transportation to bring Carl home?"

I protested, "No, I want to get him."

Stephanie screamed, "I am coming too!"

I pleaded with everyone. "I would really appreciate it if I went alone to get Carl. He and I have some fences to mend."

Everyone agreed. Dan wanted to know what the governor said about my medical license issues.

I sighed. "He was extremely apologetic, but he said he could not intervene at this point. He said that if I lost the appeal and it went to the State Board of Medicine, he might be able to help. Until then I was on my own."

Dan nodded in agreement. "It was worth asking but I think we have to respect the Governor's position. The Dagostino case is still fresh in voter's minds."

I motioned to Father Jonathan who continued his report. "Getting back to Supreme Stables. I think we have to gird our loins and go for the gusto." After a slight pause, he added. "We must have eyes and ears in that barn during quiet time. It won't be easy, but I think I can find enough time alone in the morning to set up some equipment. Joe, I need a crash course on how to get that done."

Joe nodded "I can have you ready to go with an hour or so of instruction and practice. I am sure I have what we will need in the car. We'll get to it as soon as we are done here."

Azzie and Dan were next to give their report. It was hard to believe that anything could cast a pall on the jubilation in the room, but they managed to do just that. Dan explained that my case would depend on convincing one physician member of the board of directors that I had acted appropriately. There were only three physicians on the board. Two of them were involved in the case, or the original hearing, and they therefore were excluded.

The remaining physician was I Need (my nickname for Dr. Morehead), an orthopedic surgeon. I got along well with him, but his knowledge of obstetrics, severe head trauma, and organ donation would be minimal. So, the testimony of expert witnesses would be key.

"Azzie gave me quite a war chest and so far, I have very little to show for it," Dan said dejectedly.

Azzie explained. "We aren't done yet, but Dan will explain why our task has become so difficult."

"Supreme Medical has reached out to eight of the nine expert physicians we hoped to engage. I was able to find out through the grapevine that they paid them ten times the going rate for a case review and report. Seven of the eight accepted. Now Supreme Medical has their reports."

I was optimistic. "What if those reports are favorable to me?"

Dan sighed. "It doesn't matter what they say."

Now I was pessimistic. "You are going to have to explain this better."

Dan nodded. "I told you these bylaws are strange. The hospital cannot call anyone to testify at the appeal who did not testify at the trial. We, however, are free to have experts testify on your behalf."

I grinned. "So, they wasted a lot of money for nothing?"

"No ZZ. What they did was somewhat brilliant. First of all, they can share the reports they received with the board committee provided they also share them with us. Of course, they are likely to only share ones that are unfavorable to you. But they can take snippets of the reports for Buster to use without revealing the source. Second, and perhaps most importantly, we cannot use any of the experts they have under contract. They paid them to essentially just take them off the playing field."

I was disgusted. "I told you those pricks played dirty. Now we are screwed."

Dan objected. "No one is screwed until I say so. ZZ, we just have to reach farther out in the state or consider out-of-state physicians. The one physician I have is an ER doc. Do you know Spencer O'Neil?"

I grinned. "He's a top doc. Very active in ACEP (American College of Emergency Physicians), and state EMS (Emergency Medical Services)."

"Well, that's good. He reviewed the case and is solidly on your side. He can't wait to testify. But I still want an Ob-Gyn, and someone with expertise in organ donation. I've got some feelers out and Azzie is working the phones and email. We will do our best."

I moved to close the meeting. "Let's close with a prayer."

As Father Jonathan stood, I motioned for him to sit. I led the prayer

"Dear Lord, thank you for allowing Carl to be freed of the bonds of the legal system. Thank you for removing from him the guilt over the death of Ken Harrow. Thank you for returning him to us. Please help me to forgive him and move on. Thank you for giving me the finest friends and family in the world. Finally, Lord, assist us in delivering Supreme Medical and Stable to their rightful places in hell. Amen."

CHAPTER 45

Fired Up Farms
0700 August 4

Mom grabbed a complete set of clothes. She actually grabbed regular clothes and a suit. She was so nervous that she tried to pack three pairs of underwear and socks when I stopped her.

"Mom, he won't be naked when I pick him up. I just need a shirt and a pair of pants."

"Of course, I am so happy. I can't think straight."

I walked over to her and held her tight.

"Mom, we are going to win this thing. I can just feel it. And no matter what the outcome our family will be together. And I mean together. I will be here with you, Carl, and Stephanie. We will work this out."

She was crying crocodile tears and was not able to speak. She handed me a shirt and a pair of pants. I kissed her on the cheek, and I was gone.

It was a two-hour drive to the prison. I needed that time to process my thoughts. I went over and over in my head what exactly I would say to Carl. There was no doubt that I would celebrate his newfound freedom with him. But what about our rift?

Before I could fully sort out my thoughts, I arrived at the prison. After parking the car, I proceeded through the security measures and waited. At exactly 9 AM an officer walked Carl down the hall to the waiting area. I stood and embraced him. We hugged and held and cried. After a two-minute hug, the guard cleared his throat.

"Once you sign for your belongings you are free to go."

Carl grabbed the paper and signed. We almost ran to my truck. No one spoke until we cleared the prison walls. He was first up.

"ZZ how in the hell did you work this out?"

I went through the "Dying Was Easy" call. I very carefully and ashamedly explained to him how we were drug addicts. I followed that up with our recovery and promised to help each other. Then I filled him in briefly on Joe's work that freed him, and my call to the governor. I waited for him to express his disappointment that I had been a drug addict. I was shocked when he spoke.

"ZZ, I am so proud of you beating heroin addiction. And I am proud of your friends. You folks stared down a death sentence and walked away. That took a lot of courage and determination."

"I am so ashamed that I got that low."

"Some other time ZZ, I will tell you how low I have gone. There is no need to be ashamed. I see a son who I am proud of. I see a son who loves his family, and I see a son who would have been the top harness driver in the USA if not for me. Please forgive me."

"I have thought about this a ton. You hurt me when you blackballed me from driving. Initially, I could not get past what you had done. But as time went on, I knew you did what you thought was in my best interest. I might as well tell you before you hear it. I choked a horse down last week. We both ended up on the track. There were no injuries to either of us, just a few scratches. I am ready to keep rolling but after Millions Week I need to reassess my priorities. If I ever had a son who was a harness race driver, I know I would sweat bullets with each drive."

"I too ZZ have thought this through. I did exactly like you thought. I tried to protect you. But I had no right to dictate your career. You, and only you, had the right to do that. I know we can get past this. You see, I have never told anyone this, but if I get to a point where I don't give a shit, no one can beat me. For some reason right now, I don't give a shit."

I had to pull off to a rest area. We hugged, we cried. Now two Zanders don't give a shit. I pity those who choose to oppose us. A funny thing happened at that rest area. Carl became Dad.

When we got back on the road Dad inquired about the finances for the farm and the Always Hope School. I gave him a full report but the short version would have been enough. We had to come up with $6 million by the end of Millions Week. He just shook his head in disgust.

The rest of the way home Dad quizzed me about the horses. We went over every horse in the barn and as many horses that I could think of that might enter the Millions Mile. He wanted to know about equipment, injuries, the latest times, etc. His memory was much better than mine.

We weren't done by the time we reached the farm. We were greeted by Stephanie, Mom, Azzie, and Joe.

Stephanie flew down the sidewalk and threw herself in Dad's arms.

"Who is this little beauty?" he asked with a grin.

"Your little girl, welcome home Dad!!!"

I could see on his face what exactly he was thinking. First of all, this little girl was no longer little, and she was gorgeous. She just completed an entire sentence without an expletive. How in the hell long was I away?

Mom was next. She cried and cried and tried to dry her tears. Dad just held her. No words were spoken. None were needed.

Joe struck up a chorus of "For he's a jolly good fellow" and we all joined in. Back in the house I grabbed a beer and handed one to my dad.

"Thanks, ZZ but I am taking a break from booze until this is over. Too much to do and too little time."

Mom fixed some sandwiches and Dad wanted to hear how Joe got him sprung. Joe apologized for not having a copy of the video to show him. The police had taken the copies for now. Dad was happy just to hear the story, so Joe obliged him.

"My grandfather gave me a tip on the bartender. He had some unbelievable good luck getting out of a bad situation." Joe went on to explain the gambling loss and his sudden ability to pay the money back. He went on.

"That lead me to a waitress that was not present during my first trip to the bar. She confirmed for me that you used the train to get your drinks in the pool room."

"The train?" Azzie questioned.

Dad explained the train and how he and Ken really got a kick out of their drinks coming by train.

Joe then confirmed that on the night in question, no one actually saw Ken and Carl have more than one drink. He further explained that there was ample opportunity for the drinks to be doctored at any location.

Dad added. "I remember the train, and the toast with Ken, but little else."

Joe was quick to fill in some blanks. "Not surprising, we are pretty sure you two were drugged. Learning about the train was a help but the waitress's sexual proclivity was the big break."

Joe paused a minute for effect.

"Apparently the waitress had a quickie with her boyfriend in the parking lot not too long ago."

Dad looked puzzled. "How does that tie in?"

Joe went on to detail how "Piercemaster" tried to blackmail the waitress. He explained the snooping operation that the guy was running at the Daily Double and its parking lot.

Joe continued, "I met with him, and I purchased a great video. You can't make out the perps, but it is clear on the tape that Ken was placed in the passenger seat of the truck. He appeared to be out like a light. You, Mr. Zander, were placed in the back seat of another car. You were very wobbly." There was not a sound in the room as Joe finished the story.

"The perps placed a crash dummy; you know the white one with no face and the yellow decal on it? They placed one of those in the driver's seat. Then we got to hear the only audio on the tape that was clear. As the driver got into the other car someone screamed "Make sure you hit the right tree."

"The most logical scenario that the State Police and I could reconstruct was this. Your truck's computer had been hacked to allow remote control. It was steered into a tree. Ken was killed instantly. Seconds after the accident the perps got to the accident scene. They pulled out the dummy and interrogated it. We think they ascertained the injuries that the dummy had theoretically suffered. Then they went to work to inflict them on you. Then they placed you in the vehicle. Since you were so willing to plead guilty the cops did a hasty investigation and closed the case.

In addition to the tape, we were able to locate your totaled truck. The onboard computer is being analyzed. The police are working to find the identity of the perps. Jerome, the squirrel bartender, has fled the area. The police have an ABP out for him. When they get him, they will squeeze his nuts until he sings like a Vienna Choir Boy. We may never get the identity of the person who orchestrated the plan but you never know, we could get lucky." Joe drained his beer with a gulp and accented that with a loud belch. Azzie rolled her eyes.

All my dad could say was "Holy shit."

I had already explained about the governor on the ride from the hoosegow. When Dad recovered his ability to speak, he asked about Ken's wife.

"How is she?"

I replied "Devastated as you might expect, but she was extremely happy to hear that you were not responsible. She was mad at herself for blaming you, but I told her that we all were guilty of a rush to judgment, including you."

Dad looked determined as he said "Revenge is mine sayeth the Lord. But Dear Lord as your humble servants we want to get you what is yours. And when we do, we will get enough to take care of Mrs. Harrow and her newborn son too.

CHAPTER 46

Fired Up Farms
0900 August 11

It was nice having Dad at home. This week Dan, Azzie, and I had a gazillion phone calls scheduled. We needed to plan our strategy and get our expert witnesses lined up. Normally I would have had to work those around training and barn duties, but Dad took care of all of that. In fact, Dad planned to personally train every horse that we could possibly enter in the Million Week races.

He was methodical. He carefully looked over every horse. Warmed up as many as he could, and then he took each one for their final and fastest training mile. As he got off, he passed on to Stephanie and Mom the adjustments that he wanted to make to the equipment. He also made them take explicit notes about changes he wanted to make to shoeing. Dad was nuts about shoes and horse's feet. "It all rests on those" he would say pointing from the horse's head to its chest and finally its feet.

Dan didn't have much luck finding physicians in New Jersey to testify. But he did strike gold in Philadelphia at my Alma Mater, Jefferson Medical College. Shit, that was the old name. Now it was Sidney Kimmel Medical College. Sidney or his heirs must have dumped a megafortune into Jefferson's coffers. I donated to them annually, and during my prime racing years, I thought I was quite generous. Somehow no one ever asked to name the school after me. They did put me on the cover of one Alumni magazine, so I guess I shouldn't bitch.

Regardless, Dan located two physicians to testify for me. The first, Dr. Kincaid, was actually a Phi Chi brother of mine. We both resided at 1025 Spruce Street to save money on rent. Plus, we had beer on tap 24/7. Adam Kincaid was quiet in the frat house. I was not. We got along but didn't hang around together much. He was a few years ahead of me and the upper and lower class schedules never matched up. He now ran the transplant program at Jeff Kimmel. Ok, Sidney Kimmel. He told us that he would not have been able to use any of the live organs from our patient. He might have if she had arrived at a transplant center. Our weather problems and the time we had to take to deliver the baby argued strongly against any viable organs being harvested. Adding those items to the fact that we had maxed out pressor agents, (drugs to raise blood pressure), it was his opinion that no organs were lost due to anything I did.

Celeste Maliterna was the head of Ob-Gyn. She was an attending when I was a medical student. She even let me deliver a baby when I was a third-year student. I didn't think she would remember me, but she admitted during our first call that she had a secret crush on me back then. Maybe she said she had an Orange Crush that she wanted to dump on my head. Anyway, she recognized my name from the Alumni Bulletin with my picture in my driving colors. Turns out she was a harness race fan. See when I am rolling, I am rolling.

She went over every detail of the case. She reviewed the extent of the mother's injuries, the mother's vital signs, and most importantly, the fetal monitor strips. She called me to discuss her findings.

"ZZ you are lucky you got this kid out when you did. She couldn't have lasted more than five or ten minutes longer. Had you ever done a C-section?"

"The closest I came was the second assist to you on one. Was there a problem?"

"No, I think you might have had issues had the mother survived. The autopsy pictures show a pretty sloppy C-section. But to be perfectly honest, I know I would have done the same sloppy job. Mom was moribund and the baby was in extremis. No time for nice-nice. Great work for an ER doc. It must have been the great training I gave you."

"Dr Maliterna, you have made my day. Is there any way I can repay you?"

"As a matter of fact, there is. First, please call me Celeste. Second, I always wanted to jog a harness horse."

I smiled, "Very easily arranged. Plus, it would be my family's pleasure to have you and your husband as my guests in the Owner's Club for Miracle Millions night."

"Deal!"

I hung up the phone and wandered into the living room. Dad was there watching replays of previous races. He was watching our horses and every horse that he thought might get entered in the Millions Week races. He had papers all over the place. Three empty coffee cups were on the table plus remnants of a sandwich that Mom had made him for lunch. I waited until a race he was watching finished.

"How are ya, Dad?"

"Good ZZ, how are things going for the appeal?"

"I think we will be ok in the end. We finally lined up some superstar experts. How is your preparation for Millions Week coming?"

"Slow ZZ. Being away from the races is a double-edged sword. I don't have any biases. I see what I see. But I am just not as sharp as I was."

"I'll take a "not as sharp" you over any other trainer in the world."

CHAPTER 47

Groom's Quarters
Miracle Mile Racetrack and Casino
0550 August 14

Time was short. It was only nine days until the start of Millions Week and he needed answers. No way was he going to go back to ZZ empty-handed. He lifted the mattress and found the bag containing the supplies Joe had given him. He carefully selected as much equipment as he could fit in his pants without looking suspicious. It was amazing how technological advances had been able to reduce the size of cameras and listening devices. He had to work quickly. He started in the barn at 6 AM and could not be late. Once he selected the devices he wanted, he quickly synced them to his phone. He then made his way to the barn.

"Little John, how's it hanging?" The bellowing voice of Carlton Hennessey, lead trainer for Supreme Stables, jolted Father Jonathan who had his back toward the front of the stall.

"If you scare the shit out of me again, I will pull it out and beat you to death with it."

"Funny big boy. You are in a little early today, what's up?"

Father Jonathan was thinking. Well, I have a bunch of cameras to plant around here, and I was casing the joint. Instead, he said, "I woke up early and figured why not get an early start."

"Well, better than being late, but don't make a habit of it. We frown down on anyone, I mean anyone, being in the barn alone. You never know who may want to drug our horses to make it look like we cheat."

It was all Father Jonathan could do not to vomit. He quickly changed the subject. "No problem, who are you training today?"

Carlton handed him a schedule with the horse's names, times, and the person who would be training or jogging them. Say what you want, but these people were organized.

The morning went quickly, almost too quickly. Every time he had a free minute, he scoped out the best places to put cameras. But the only place he got set up was the tack room. It was a busy barn and people were going in and out all the time. Later in the morning, he found himself with ten minutes alone in the barn. That was enough time to finish deploying the equipment. Carlton was walking in as he was leaving. He said goodbye to Carlton and quickly departed for his groom's quarters.

He was pleased with the quality of the pictures and the sound. He had a good look at the barn and could hear reasonably well. If there was anything amiss in there, he would know it in the next few days. He found a bag of stale potato chips, grabbed a beer, and connected his laptop. He really hated the small screen on his phone.

He sipped his beer as he watched the barn activity. He saw or heard nothing unusual. Not that he expected to. He really thought that his biggest finds would occur during quiet time. He went to the bathroom to be sure he could watch for the next few hours without interruption. He knew it was overkill because he was recording this, but he really wanted to watch live. There was a knock on the door as he exited the bathroom, and he opened the door. As he did so, the door blasted completely open, and he ended up on his ass on the floor. Before he could say or do anything, he was grabbed by three men, secured by zip ties to his wrists and ankles, and gagged.

He recognized one of the men who appeared to be the leader of the pack. It was Kris "Knuckles" Markovich. He was the head of security for Supreme Medical Center. I had mentioned him during the discussion the other night and had pictures of him and Deuce. Father Jonathan watched as Knuckles looked at the laptop and scrolled through the various camera feeds. Knuckles breathed heavily into his lip mike.

"Looks like four cameras Carlton. One in the tack room, one at each end of the barn, and one somewhere in the middle." Father

Jonathan could not hear the response, but he did hear Knuckle's reply a few minutes later.

"You got three, the only one left is the one in the center of the barn. It's just about near the center of the hallway, in front of stall ten."

A few more minutes went by and the screen on the laptop went blank.

Knuckles declared, "All clear."

He packed the laptop and phone and got into Father Jonathan's face. "Now we are going to stand you up and remove the cuffs. But before we do that, we are going to attach these taser wires to your back. Have you ever been tased?"

No answer.

The wires were attached.

Knuckles continued, "It's not pleasant."

"What do you want?" Father Jonathan inquired as the gag was removed.

"We want to ask you a few questions but we don't want to do it here. If you want to get out of this in one piece, you will walk out of here quietly and get into the van."

"If I don't want to be quiet?"

"Then we will tase you at twice the usual dose. You see, I get these made special. Once you are unconscious, we will put you in the van and take you somewhere to question you."

"What if someone sees? There will be questions."

"Just a thieving groom who resisted proper arrest. I have a warrant here."

"Bogus, of course!"

"Yeah, but good enough to fool any dimwitted horsemen who might happen to see something."

"I'll go quietly."

"Wise choice, Little John."

They removed the ties and all four men walked quietly to the van. Once inside the van, the zip ties were reapplied and secured to the van seat belt. Little John's right hand was used to obtain fingerprints.

"Do I get a hood? Like in the middle east? Where are you taking me?"

Knuckles grinned. "You get a gag, but no hood. You are going where all pieces of shit go."

Little John's arms and legs shook violently. His back arched involuntarily as the taser discharged.

"I always get a kick out of that. It makes me think like I am a doctor using the paddles on some dude." Knuckles laughed.

CHAPTER 48

Krenshaw Municipal Sewage Plant
1400 August 14

Father Jonathan had little recall of the tasing. As he came to, he found himself tied to a chair with his arms in front. He was not gagged nor hooded. The smell was overwhelming. He knew that people often shit themselves when tased, but this smell was much worse than anything he had ever created in his life. As he opened his eyes, he noticed he was neck-deep in brown frothy water mixed with pungent turds.

"Hey asshole, are you awake?" The voice was not familiar. It belonged to one of the two men sitting in lounge chairs above the tank. Knuckles was not there.

"Get me the hell out of here. What is this place?" yelled Father Johnathan.

"We told you we were taking you to a place where pieces of shit go because you are a piece of shit. This is the sewage treatment plant." Guffaws erupted from above.

"What do you want?"

"Tell us who you are working for, and we let you go."

Father Jonathan pondered the question. Sure, I am Father Jonathan, a Catholic priest on special assignment with a mafia dude and a cosmetic diva to save ZZ's horse farm and school for special kids. Even if he wanted to tell them, who would believe it?

"I am not working for anyone."

A large bucket of shit and brown water was dumped on his bald head. He gagged as the swill ran down his face and soaked his beard.

"Wrong answer asshole, try again. Why were you bugging the barn?"

"I work alone. I bugged the barn to try to get inside information that I could use to bet."

Another bucket found its target. This time Father Jonathan vomited violently.

"We got all day pal, but I don't think your guts will hold up."

Father Jonathan heard a cell phone ring and barely heard someone say that the fingerprints were traced to Jonathan Winters aka Little John. The last address was Pittsburgh.

"Hey asshole, are you a Steelers fan?"

"What the difference does that make? "Father Johnathan screamed.

"Where did you live in Pittsburgh?"

"Why?"

Another bucket dumped its fetid contents on Little John's head.

"We ask the questions. Do you want to get out of there? If so, wise up."

"I went to Duquesne University." He waited for another pail of fun but none came. In fact, he could no longer see the guys in the chairs. He did hear the rotors start-up that mixed up the decomposing gaga. He thought for sure one would cut him but it missed by inches. The rotor did create waves that shoved poopy water over his head every thirty seconds. This went on for the next two hours.

He hadn't noticed the wire that protruded from the back of his shirt and ended at the top of the tank. Not that he could have done anything about it. Just as the rotor stopped the taser knocked him out cold. The next thing he knew he was sitting on a bench at a bus stop. He was covered in sewage, and his own vomit. People stared at him, but no one was in a hurry to join him on the bench. In fact, most of the riders quickly found alternative means of transportation.

At least ten people turned him down before a kind soul agreed to make the phone call that Little John begged to have placed. The kind soul was upwind. She offered to place the call but wisely refused to let Little John touch her phone.

The Good Samaritan inquired. "Is ZZ there?"

"No, who is this?" Azzie replied.

Father Jonathan screamed at the Good Samaritan, "Ask for Azzie."

"Is Azzie there?"

"This is Azzie."

"Do you know a guy named Little John?"

"Yes. Why? Who are you?"

Little John worried that Azzie would hang up, so he screamed, "Azzie come get me at 7th and Waterford Streets."

Azzie recognized the voice but wanted more information. The Good Samaritan felt she had done enough good deeds for one day and ended the call. The wind had shifted, and she was disgusted. She had no way to know that Little John had been treated to a sewage spa treatment. She just thought he was a smelly homeless person and she had enough. Twenty minutes later Joe and Azzie showed up in Stephanie's pickup truck. Joe jumped out.

"You look like shit, and smell worse than that. What the hell happened?"

"Long story, let me get in the truck and I will tell you on the way back to the farm."

"No way, Jose`. Stephanie would kill me if you got inside that truck. Climb in the truck bed and don't touch more than you have to."

Azzie rolled the window down just long enough to let out a forceful "PU." The window went back up.

Father Jonathan reluctantly crawled into the bed of the immaculate white Toyota Tundra.

Back at the barn, they hosed him off and gave him some soap that they used to bathe the horses. It took a while, but they eventually got him clean enough to get into the house to take a shower. I got home as Father Jonathan walked into the house. Once I knew he was ok, I laughed my ass off as did Joe and Azzie. Father Jonathan did not see the humor we saw. A few minutes later, Stephanie walked into the house and proclaimed, "I smell shit." We all, including Father Jonathan, laughed. Stephanie quickly stopped laughing when we told her that we took her truck to pick him up. She ran out to sniff her truck. Father Jonathan took a long hot shower and joined us in the den.

"Who needs a drink?" Joe inquired as he got behind the bar.

"Give me a bottle." Said Father Jonathan with a laugh.

"Seriously?"

"Nah, just a good martini. We have a lot to discuss."

After dinner, the dishes were cleared, fresh coffee was poured, and the meeting began. Azzie was in charge as usual. She looked at Father Jonathan and proclaimed "Father, your day stunk the most, why don't you go first."

"Very funny. How long am I going to have to listen to this harassment?"

"Probably the rest of your life," I said giggling.

"Ok. Ok." Father Jonathan sipped his coffee, took a deep breath, and continued.

"As you know, they caught me setting up cameras in the barn. No one said it, but I suspect Knuckles has 24/7 surveillance in there. I know no one saw me, but bammo, two hours later I was in deep shit." (Guffaws abounded).

"What, other than tasing you and dipping you in crap, did they do or want?" asked Dad.

"That's what I can't figure. They fingerprinted me and took me to the sewage treatment plant. They kept asking me who I worked for. After about an hour of that, they turned the rotors on so the waves hit me every thirty seconds. After a couple hours of that, they tased me. I woke up and called from the bus stop. That's all I know."

Joe summed up. "Ok, they let you go without much damage. So, they don't think anything serious is wrong with their operation. Thank God our security measures worked. You were smart to post those things on Facebook about your time at Duquesne University but to delete any references to being a priest. Priests don't often seek employment in stables. If they had uncovered any information connecting you with ZZ, you might be dead."

"But I am convinced that they are dirty."

I added, "I am 100% convinced that they are, but we have zero chance of getting any information out of that barn now."

After a spirited discussion, the group decided that Father Jonathan should not go back. He should stay here, out of sight. He was tasked with researching the sudden rise of Supreme Stables from mediocrity to being the top stable in all of harness racing.

Father Jonathan inquired about how long Supreme Stables had been dominating harness racing.

Dad answered, "Somewhere around two to three years. Four years ago, we were on top. Supremes had horses for about two years before then but they were just average players. They went through trainers like ZZ gnawing on fresh corn on the cob. Then one day they settled on Carlton Hennessey. Overnight their fortunes changed."

"What do you know about Hennessey?" Father Jonathan wanted to know.

"I first noticed that he seemed competent, ran a tight ship. I thought their newfound success was mostly due to him."

"And?" I asked.

"Then I talked to some connections I had in Canada. They had nicknamed him 'Carl the chemist.' They said he was dirty, but no one could ever prove it."

Father Jonathan took copious notes.

I took the floor. "Tomorrow is the final appeal with the board of directors. We have a panel of three board members including one physician, although he is an orthopedic surgeon. We are permitted to present expert testimony, and then we have to cross our fingers. If we win, we are done. I only need to see the lead judge at the track and my license is restored. If we lose, we can still sue through the courts. But that will take months and I am suspended until it is over."

CHAPTER 49

Fired Up Farms
0800 August 15

Father Jonathan was up early Friday and pecked away at his computer. Azzie and I went to the appeal. Dad, Mom, and Stephanie had been at the track since way before dawn. The coffee was hot, the house was quiet, and Father Jonathan was making progress. He was able to find out that three years ago Supreme Stables had 20 wins with a stable of 13 horses. The following year they had 100 wins with 15 horses. Last year they tallied 700 wins with 200 horses.

He already knew that they were particularly good at claiming horses, but the actual figures shocked him. Eighty-five percent of their claims won their first time out. Sixty percent of those wins happened with the horses up in class. The data was phenomenal and unbelievably good.

Somehow Supreme Stables was able to claim horses for say $10,000 and then put them in the following week for $15,000. The difference was that 60% of the time their horses won even though they were racing tougher competition. How did they do that in a week? Training and equipment changes don't let you move up that fast and consistently.

Father Jonathan's thoughts were interrupted by Dad letting himself in the front door.

"Hello Padre, did you solve the riddle yet?"

"No, Mr. Zander. Not quite. But I do have some data on Supreme Stables that shows astronomical improvement over the past two years."

Dad looked over the printout for a few minutes and then shook his head.

"Yep, sounds about right. The better they did, the worse the rest of us did. There can only be one winner in each race."

"Other than PEDS (performance-enhancing drugs), can you think of any other reason why they improved so much. "

"Well to a certain extent success breeds success. As you make more money you have more money to spend on horses and equipment. That adds to the momentum. But it would never explain this turnaround."

"Alright, I will dig deeper."

"Good luck Padre. I have to get cracking on figuring out who we are going to enter next week. All entries for the big races have to be in tomorrow along with the entry fee. The entry fee is non-refundable. Once you enter you must race or forfeit the cash."

"Are the entry fees expensive?"

"Most of them are $50,000 to $200,000. We will have about $500,000 invested, if not more."

Father Jonathan whistled and added. "Wow, you better get studying."

Dad retreated to the den where he had his computer, papers, and war room set up.

CHAPTER 50

Executive Boardroom

Supreme Medical Center

1000 August 15

I held the door to the boardroom open for Drs, O'Neil, Kincaid, and Maliterna. Dan and Azzie had left breakfast a little early to get set up in the boardroom. During breakfast, Dan laid out the procedures to be followed for today and his strategy. He had explained that this was a little different from the "trial" in that the three members who had to make the decision had been given the minutes of the "trial" in advance. In addition, they had been given the hospital's list of charges and the medical staff's reasons that each charge should stand. Finally, they received a copy of the written statements of our defense witnesses. All of this had been submitted and was to be reviewed prior to this morning to expedite the proceeding.

I looked at the people seated across the table from us and recognized most of them. From my left to right there sat Buster, Deuce, Eat A Ton Shapiro, I Need, Penelope Bradshaw, Mason Upton, and three others that I did not recognize. Penelope and Mason were board members who had been appointed to the committee by the board chair. Penelope was in her sixties and was a fixture at every significant social gathering south of New York and East of Philadelphia. All of our research indicated that she likely would be pretty solidly in Deuce's court and therefore would need a lot of convincing to sway her. Mason Upton ran a local trucking company. He appeared to be a straight shooter and we had no idea how he was leaning.

I whispered to Dan. "What the hell are Buster and Deuce doing here?"

"They are here ex officio."

"English please."

"By virtue of their elected or appointed positions, they are permitted to attend all board meetings and sub-board meetings."

"So, they have to stay?"

"Yes."

"Who are the other three stooges at the end of the table?"

"I don't know but we will soon find out."

Eat A Ton rapped a gavel and called the meeting to order. He read off some rules to be followed. For some odd reason, he looked at me when he read the rules on decorum. Prick. I was a good boy and just smiled at him. And truthfully, I think that pissed him off. Good start.

Buster started to read the charges when Dan objected. One of Dan's worries, which he shared at breakfast, was that the hospital would try to slow walk the proceedings. That was an effort to try to have their topics get disproportionate time. The idea was to clog up the proceedings with trivia and put a time constraint on any deliberation. They had a 3 PM deadline. The less new information the board members received the less likely they were to overturn the "trial."

Dan stood. "Sir, to my knowledge these are truncated proceedings. Reading of the charges is superfluous. And as a point of order, I would like to know the identity, and purpose in being here, of the three individuals at the end of your table."

Buster was taken aback. "I just thought that we should refresh everyone's memory of the very serious charges. The three distinguished individuals at the end of the table are the expert witnesses the hospital intends to call to expound our position."

"Sir, the hospital cannot call any witnesses. They did not use any outside witnesses in the trial. The testimony of the medical staff members who did participate in the trial has been included in the information shared with the committee. In addition, the reading of the charges that are in the record or other tactics you might employ to waste time detract from the sanctimony of these proceedings."

Penelope raised her hand. "I would like to hear what the hospital witnesses have to say."

Dan quickly responded, "So would I have during the 'trial.' But according to the bylaws my client was not permitted to have representation at the 'trial.'"

He paused.

"And according to the bylaws, the hospital was permitted to have expert witnesses testify at the 'trial.' However, the only witnesses that can testify at this appeal are ones that either testified for the hospital at the 'trial' or ones that testify for the physician charged. The hospital in its haste to punish my client did not call any expert witnesses at the trial. Therefore, the hospital witnesses can be excused."

That caused a major discussion at the other table. Dan had his stopwatch out, and at the five-minute mark, he rose.

"Sir, time is wasting. Please rule on the witnesses."

Eat A Ton looked defeated. "The witnesses for the hospital are excused."

Buster then listed the charges to be reviewed. Any charges dropped or admitted to were not included. That only left three charges to be reviewed.

Wrongful death of Cynthia Walker

Inappropriate C section

Loss of potentially donated organs

Buster droned on:

"In regard to the wrongful death of Cynthia Walker, the hospital contends that had she been transported directly from the scene to a trauma center that she may have survived."

Dan interjected. "Our expert, Spencer O'Neil, disagrees in his written opinion."

Penelope jumped in. "But the hospital experts thought that immediate transfer would have given her a chance."

Dan smiled. "Thank you, Ms. Bradshaw. Since you have broached this subject that permits my client to allow his witnesses to answer. Dr O'Neil?"

Spencer cleared his throat. "Mam, this was a tragic case but not a difficult one to analyze from the perspective of this proceeding. This patient had severe, and I underline the word severe, head trauma. She had brain matter exuding from her wounds. She was a Glasgow Coma Scale 3. That is dead, mam. The Glasgow Coma Scale starts at 3 and goes to 15. At 3 you are dead. This patient was dead."

Penelope mumbled. "No further questions."

Buster read the next charge. "Loss of donated organs." Then he launched into a detailed discussion about the benefits of organ donation. I think I just figured out why Buster was so passionate about organ donation. The way he drank his liver was about to explode at any minute. He wanted to make sure he could find a replacement. Dan's voice brought me back to reality.

"I object," Dan shouted.

Eat A Ton glared back at Dan. "State your reason for objection."

Dan quickly responded. "Everyone knows the value of donated organs; the hospital is dragging out the proceedings again."

Buster knew he was busted. "Ok we all stipulate that donated organs are valuable, and in this case, Dr. Zander lost valuable organs due to his incompetence"

Dan jumped to his feet. "We do not stipulate a thing. I do vehemently object to Dr. Hyman's use of the term incompetence. We call Dr. Kincaid."

Buster walked over in front of Dr. Kincaid and placed his shaking hands on our table. "Dr. Kincaid, have you ever harvested donated organs from a patient with injuries as severe as Cynthia Walker?"

"Yes, I have."

Buster nodded. "Could you have harvested organs from Cynthia Walker?"

"Possibly, had she arrived in my trauma center with her organs being perfused."

Dan interrupted. "But she was in the field, and an expeditious trauma center transfer was not possible due to weather. Could you still have harvested her organs if it took another forty minutes to get to your facility?"

Kincaid calmly replied. "No. By that time there was no chance."

All three board members looked down.

Buster brought them all back to focus. "Our last charge is the inappropriate C-section performed by Dr. Zander."

Buster droned on with the description from the trial. Dan was unable to protest because it was allowed in testimony.

Dan finally did find his voice. "Our expert would like to give testimony."

Buster objected. "No need, we have their written notes."

Mason Upton raised his hand and was recognized by Eat A Ton. "I want to hear from the expert witness."

Eat A Ton relented. "Dr. Maliterna, please proceed."

Celeste launched. "Given the moribund condition of the mother it was more appropriate to focus on attempting to save the child. The child was about 38 weeks gestation, which made her almost full-term. But to me, the crux of the C-section charge lies in the fetal monitoring strips that were obtained on arrival to the ED. They showed severe fetal distress. Every second that child stayed in that womb was a second that child was not getting vital oxygen. Although Dr. Zander had never performed a C-section, he did a commendable job of getting that baby out."

"Listen, sweetie," Buster interrupted in a very condescending tone. "I was delivering babies while you were still making doo doo in your diaper. I know obstetrics. Had she been brought directly to the trauma center the section could have been done by better trained and more appropriately credentialed physicians."

Maliterna's veins in her neck bulged and she cut loose. "Come on, Grandpa. I grant you that I may have been in diapers when you started practicing. Now I am delivering babies while you are making doo doo in your diaper. It's called continuing medical education. You ought to get some. But even a doctor as out of touch as you has to understand that the outcome was excellent. There would have been no better outcome at a trauma center as far as the baby was concerned."

Both sides shouted objections and epithets. Eat A Ton broke the gavel pounding it on the desk.

Dan screamed above the din. "Any further questions for Dr. Maliterna?"

Upton responded. "No further questions for her but I do have a question that needs to be asked."

Eat A Ton tried to hold the pieces of his gavel together. After a few seconds, he gave up and acknowledged Mr. Upton. "Please proceed."

Upton rocked back in his chair and cupped his hands behind his head. "Not being of a medical background sometimes has its blessings. In my mind, I can see that a key point in this unfortunate case was that the patient was not flown directly to a trauma center. Had she been flown there Dr. Zander never would have been placed in the position he was.

Dan looked a little spooked. "Your point?"

Upton continued. "I occasionally fly in a helicopter for business. I have had a few instances where the pilots said this or that about the weather and wanted to delay or divert. On one particular occasion, I had a severe time deadline to meet for a bid for a lucrative contract. I demanded we continue on when the pilot wanted to ground. We made it safely. My point is that I think that the prospect of helicopter transfer was abandoned too early. Dr. Zander should have been more forceful in his request. Maybe he *was* interested somewhat in impressing his staff."

I began to rise to speak when I was pushed down in my seat by Dr. O'Neil.

O'Neil offered. "I would like to answer your question, sir."

Upton agreed. "Please do."

O'Neil nodded. "Thank you. I have spoken with the pilot for Air Angel, (the helicopter service used), who was on that night. It might behoove all to know that the pilot of the helicopter is the sole person deciding whether weather conditions are suitable for air evacuation. He or she is not told anything about the patient. Their decision is based solely upon the safety of the flight. The system is set up so that patient information does not bias their thinking. The pilot who made the decision not to fly that night flew helicopters in Iraq and has been with Air Angel for four years. Her record is impeccable. According to her, the weather conditions that night were not safe. She refused to put her crew and aircraft in a dangerous situation. So, she declined the flight. When I told her about the patient her response was this:

O'Neil applied his reading glasses and read from a paper he pulled from his coat pocket. "That information would have changed nothing. Dangerous weather is dangerous weather. I can't risk four lives to try to save one."

O'Neil slowly removed his reading glasses and finished his remarks. "Dr. Hyman, on his own, contacted the dispatcher for the ambulance service and demanded that they take the patient directly to the trauma center by ground. Dr. Hyman is not a medical command physician. The laws in New Jersey do not permit him to order medics to do anything. They can only take orders from a licensed medical command physician. Dr. Hyman had no legal or medical authority to countermand the orders of a duly licensed and qualified medical command physician such as Dr. Zander. The only time a non-medical command physician can intervene in the field is if they are physically present, take full responsibility for their actions, and accompany the patient to the hospital in the ambulance. Dr. Hyman did none of those."

Buster exploded. "Look you little shit. What those medics do at times in the field is atrocious and wrong. This time I gave them an opportunity to make a difference for this poor unfortunate victim and they ignored me. Look at the outcome."

O'Neill ignored the "little shit" slur. "Based upon the condition of the patient it is my assessment that her chances of surviving were negligible at best. Once direct helicopter transfer was not possible, she was doomed. The medics and Dr. Zander heroically kept her alive to save her baby and organs. Unfortunately, by the time the baby was delivered, the patient had died, and her organs were no longer viable."

Dr. Maliterna jumped into the fray. "I can state with certainty that had she been transported directly to the trauma center by ambulance that night, as Dr. Hyman wanted, her baby would have died."

Upton appeared satisfied. "Thank you, doctors, I think I understand the situation much better now."

I saw Azzie exit the room out of the corner of my eye. Too much coffee?

Dan stood. "I have one last witness to call."

Eat A Ton pounded the table with his fist due to his broken gavel. "Out of order, you listed three, and we received testimony from three. The fourth cannot be used. You should have asked them to put their testimony in a report like the others."

Dan just stood and said nothing. The door opened and Azzie pranced into the room holding a pink blanket.

Dan proclaimed, "Our final witness is Zee Zee Walker."

Eat A Ton screamed, "Out of order!"

Dan ignored him and continued. "She doesn't have much to say but I think you all can appreciate the value of her presence. Yes, her grandparents who are raising her named her Zee Zee in honor of Dr.

Zander. They credit him with allowing Zee Zee to live in spite of all odds. They and our other witnesses know that many ER physicians would not have had the guts to attempt a lifesaving C-section. Thanks to Dr. Zander, the Walkers have two granddaughters to raise and a fond remembrance of their son and daughter-in-law."

I Need finally spoke. He had yet to ask a question or offer an opinion. I had wondered if he was sleeping. "I for one am ready to deliberate."

Eat A Ton questioned the others. "Ms. Bradshaw? Mr. Upton? Do you need any more time or information?"

"No." "No."

They adjourned to the private dining area off the conference room. Azzie took me out to meet the Walkers. Mrs. Walker kissed me, and Mr. Walker saluted me. They were both crying. So was Azzie. Zee Zee and I were the only two dry ones.

"I am sorry for the loss of your son and daughter-in-law," I told them.

Mrs. Walker was quick to respond. "It has been extremely difficult, but this little package and her sister keep us busy. That is good."

Our conversation was interrupted by Eat A Ton screaming for us to get back in the room. I bid farewell to the Walkers and kissed Zee Zee on the forehead. I really had to whiz but Eat A Ton was going wild.

He started to read the charges again but I Need cut him off.

"Haven't we heard them enough! I, for one, am embarrassed to have to sit here and learn just how low our medical staff has fallen. These charges were ridiculous. In light of the testimony heard today, the notes of the trial, and the written proffers of the witnesses I vote to dismiss the three remaining charges."

Eat A Ton objected. "But doctor …."

I Need was having none of it. "Look here you twit; I told you I had enough. But since you interrupted me, I further move that all previous charges against Dr. Zander be dismissed. Even the ones he stipulated to!" I Need's face was beet red.

Eat A Ton turned to Bradshaw. "Ms. Bradshaw, how do you vote?"

Bradshaw looked in Buster's direction. "I vote to uphold all three charges as written. I feel Dr. Zander is a dangerous physician and should not be part of our stellar medical staff."

Eat A Ton shifted his attention to Upton. "Mr. Upton the ball is in your court."

"As I mentioned during the appeal, my big concern was whether or not Dr. Zander interfered with the transport to the trauma center that Dr. Hyman had arranged. It is clear to me that Dr Zander did interfere."

I was deflated. Dan just stood with his mouth open, there were no words coming out. How in the hell could this guy rule against us?

Upton continued. "Fortunately, Dr. Zander had the courage and tenacity to do what he thought was right in spite of overwhelming pressure from his medical staff president. That is the same medical staff president that I saw consuming numerous adult beverages at the country club on the very night of the accident."

Eat A Ton rapped the end of the broken gavel on the table. "Out of order, out of order. I insist on order! Mr. Upton please!"

"Piss on you pal. I have watched you and your buddy Hofecker ruin numerous physicians over the years. I was moved by the testimony of the experts we have here today. They convinced me that Dr. Zander acted appropriately. Thanks only to Dr. Zander that baby we just saw got a chance at life. I also vote to have all previous charges against Dr. Zander stricken. If he would have acted with anything except malice, considering how he was treated, I would have to question his metal."

There was silence until Dan spoke up.

"We thank the panel for their diligence and courage."

I Need bolted for the door and was gone before I could thank him. I had to shake Upton's hand.

"Thanks."

"No, thank you, Dr. Zander. I Hope you elect to stay on here although I would understand if you elected to leave."

"I am not sure what I am going to do but you opened a lot of doors for me. I will never forget it."

CHAPTER 51

Fired Up Farms
1430 August 15

Father Jonathan looked for everything he could find out about Carlton Hennesey, the trainer for Supreme Stables. Nothing stood out. He was successful in Canada but nowhere near as successful as he had been here. The fines and suspensions he received from the Canadian Trotting and US Trotting Association were routine for a large stable. He only had one post-race-positive drug test three years ago. Despite having many more horses racing, he had none in the past two years. That was a little odd. Odd, but not damning.

Out of boredom from finding next to nothing he decided to search Supreme Medical. He sorted through hundreds of feel-good articles the hospital had promoted. Articles proclaiming that Supreme Medical was rated number one in anal itch treatment by the Society to Prevent Anal Itch etc. Eventually, he found one that intrigued him. Supreme Medical was for-profit. Five years ago, it was a struggling non-profit that was purchased for a song. Supreme Medical Associates gained control by assuming the debt of the hospital. Further research revealed that Supreme Medical Associates was owned and controlled by none other than Thomas Earhardt Hofecker II.

Father Jonathan kept digging. The first two years as a for-profit, they barely broke even. However, the last three years were quite lucrative. Wow, old man Hofecker was smoking on all cylinders. His concentration was interrupted by his cell phone singing "On Eagles Wings," one of his favorite hymns.

"Hello, this is John."

Azzie screamed, "We Won! We Won! I will be home around 3 PM."

She hung up before Father Jonathan could get a word in. In a few minutes, the peace and quiet was interrupted again by Joe barreling in the door.

"Boom, boom, boom! ZZ wins again, going away!"

Father Jonathan stood up and they high fived. Then they retreated to the kitchen for an adult beverage. Azzie arrived at the same time as Mom and Stephanie. Mom wanted to start dinner, but Azzie interrupted her.

"Let's order some pizza. I'm too tired, and too happy to help you cook."

They ordered pizzas to be delivered. Joe insisted on anchovies on at least one. "I love anchovies and so does ZZ. Where is the guest of honor?"

"ZZ asked me to give you the details of the appeal and he asked me to apologize to all of you for his absence. He has a date with Jenny. You know Dan did forbid any contact with her until the appeal was over." Azzie explained.

"Mr. Gadoonga must be really hungry by now." Stephanie blurted out causing everyone to study their feet.

"Who is this Mr. Gadoonga? We should invite him over. We have plenty of pizza coming." Mom was clueless.

Azzie quickly changed the subject. "Forget it, let's get a drink and I'll share the details of a great victory. Dan has another pressing case. He will try to join us later."

Azzie's blow-by-blow description was interrupted only by occasional screams of joy and back-slapping. The pizza arrived and they all dug in.

Joe inquired "Who is racing tonight? I feel lucky. I am ready to make a big score."

Dad broke his bubble. "Maybe tomorrow, Joe. We have nothing in tonight. I have most horses racing tomorrow to be tight for Millions Miles next Saturday."

Joe moved on. "OK Padre, what do you have to show for a day in front of that computer screen?"

Father Jonathan shared the information with the group that he had reviewed with Dad.

Joe's speech was garbled by a mouth full of pizza, "pretty damn suspicious."

Father Jonathan responded. "I agree, but I can't connect the dots just yet. I did however find out that Supreme Medical's financial health improved in a parallel time frame to the Stable"

Joe laughed. "How do you drug a hospital to do better?"

Father Jonathan said he needed a little more time to research Deuce.

Azzie forgot that she promised to call Juicy Lucy. She had wanted to be informed of the outcome of the hearing. Azzie punched a button on her cell phone.

"Lucy, this is Azzie. We won! Sorry, I forgot to call you earlier."

"Thanks, but I already heard the good news."

"You did?"

"The hospital is buzzing and my boss is seething."

"That's good to hear, I just wanted to thank you. Your help was invaluable."

"No problem. Is ZZ there? I'd like to congratulate him."

"No, he's out on a date."

"With that bitch Jenny?"

"Lucy, I will leave that for you and ZZ to discuss."

"I guess you are right. That guy rings my bell if you know what I mean. I don't understand why he would date Hofecker's niece."

"What?"

"Jenny Rich is Deuce's niece. You didn't know?"

"I didn't know, and neither does ZZ. Is there anything else he should know?"

"Dah, yeah! The rumor is that she shot and killed a guy in Florida. Deuce got her a hot shit attorney who convinced the prosecutor not to press charges. After that, she moved here and changed her name."

"ZZ had absolutely no idea."

"Well, you better tell him. And remind him that my wedding is coming up."

Azzie thought silently for a few seconds. "This Lucy IS Juicy, and she has a thing for ZZ. Not just a thing. She is getting married and wants ZZ to be her last fling. She smiled and said into the phone. "I will tell him."

Just then the ramifications of what she just heard registered in her brain. Azzie screamed, "Code Blue, all hands-on deck."

Everyone gathered around as Azzie announced what she had learned.

Stephanie's face was scarlet. "That bitch pretended to know nothing about the races and never mentioned any relationship to Deuce. She is in this up to her big tits, and ZZ is in danger."

Azzie dialed my cell phone and heard it ringing in her purse. She had held it for me during the hearing and forgot to give it back.

Father Jonathan shrieked. "Look at this. A computer programmer was shot to death by a Gennifer Poorman."

Father Jonathan shared a link so they could read with him. The victim was a computer programmer in charge of IT for The Competition Integrity Committee. In response to numerous reports of horse and human athletic doping, congress created the committee. The purpose was to standardize, and centralize, all drug testing for competition. Professional sports, the Olympics, and all horse racing would be analyzed by a single entity. The idea was to do all of the testing in one lab in one location and fund it with hundreds of millions of dollars. The intent was to detect even the slightest amount of all performance-enhancing drugs.

Aaron Jurovich was the head of IT and was mainly responsible for cybersecurity. While in Florida he had an affair with an ER nurse, Gennifer Poorman. Somehow, Gennifer found out Jurovich was married and was due to complete his duties soon in Florida. She had heard that he planned to return to his wife in Colorado and she confronted him. During the confrontation, Jurovich was shot in the pelvis and head and died. Poorman claimed he assaulted her, and she shot him in self-defense. The article indicated that very graphic pictures of the injuries Gennifer Poorman suffered swayed the prosecutor that the self-defense claim had merit. She was never charged.

Azzie suddenly screamed, "Oh shit! Juicy Lucy was right!"

All eyes turned to her. She motioned for everyone to get behind her so they could see her screen. On it was a blown-up picture of Gennifer Poorman. Azzie used an app she had to change the hair color, lengthen the hair, and add glasses. Gennifer Poorman transferred instantly to Jenny Rich. The room was filled with gasps.

Joe barked out orders. "Father Jonathan and Azzie, go to Jenny's apartment. If it looks like they are there, call me, but don't go in. Carl and Mrs. Zander go to the hospital. ZZ's allowed in now and he may be meeting her there. Look for his truck in all lots. Stephanie, do you have any idea where they liked to go out?"

Stephanie shook her head. "No, but I will drive around to a few restaurants that ZZ talks about."

Joe turned to address the group as he exited the front door. "I will go to the police and see if I can get some traffic cam footage after ZZ left the trial. Remember everyone, if you find them, stay back until we figure out what to do."

CHAPTER 52

Jenny's Apartment
1600 August 15

"Hey ZZ, you won big today. Got anything else big? I like big." Jenny teased.

"Well little girl, I do have a big bag of candy." I joined in the charade.

"What do I have to do to get some?" The teasing intensified.

"Come here you little vixen."

Jenny stood up and walked to the door. "It's a nice afternoon, why don't we take your big bag of candy to the lake?"

"It is difficult to walk with a big bag of candy." I protested.

"Well waddle for now then, we'll fix that problem shortly."

I could hardly wait as Jenny grabbed a bottle of wine, a blanket, and a large bag.

"What's in there?" I inquired.

"Sex toys!" Jenny giggled.

On the way to the lake, Jenny reviewed some very explicit sexual desires that she was hoping to have fulfilled. I couldn't take too much more and I offered to stop at the Marriot that we just passed.

"Take it easy ZZ, I will make this worth your while."

It seemed like an eternity, but we finally arrived at the lake. I pulled into a parking space, but Jenny just shook her head.

"Do you want an audience or just a good time? I don't like to perform for crowds. How about we go to the other, more deserted, side of the lake?"

"

Mr. G did not want to hear it, but he was holstered. I found a very secluded spot and shut the car off. Instantly Jenny sprung Mr. G from his bondage and did her best to give him a good view of her tonsils. It had been a while, so that event didn't last too long. Jenny removed her clothes and grabbed the blanket and wine from the back seat. She spread the blanket on the grass under a large oak tree. She opened the container and offered me a large glass.

"Hey, I have to drive us home, maybe a smaller glass?"

"C'mon ya wussy, we will be here quite a while." Jenny pouted as she poured herself a generous glass. We clinked glasses and I took a big, long drink. Jenny offered a toast to my victory, and I took another big gulp. Another toast to the upcoming races and my glass was empty. Jenny said she had to pee. She jumped up and ran behind the tree.

All of a sudden it felt like a truck hit me. My head was spinning, and I could not focus. I tried to scream but the best I could do was whimper and drool. Jenny returned from behind the tree and sat calmly sipping her wine. I told Mr. G that we had been drugged. That bitch Jenny did it. Then I passed out.

Jenny worked quickly. She pulled out the bag containing the fentanyl, and the tourniquet. She fired up a massive dose and sucked it into the syringe. She placed the tourniquet on my arm and thumped my vein to make it pop up. Then she inserted the needle. Effortless job for an ER nurse. She paused before she pushed the plunger.

"ZZ, I don't know if you can hear me but if you can please note that this is…"

Before she could finish the sentence, Jenny was blindsided by a blitzing linebacker. Her attacker called her a fucking whore and proceeded to pummel her face mercilessly. Jenny tried to fight back but she was no match for her opponent, even though Jenny was much taller. The little one had too much power. Jenny saw stars and planned for the worst when the beating stopped. Head wounds oozed blood into her eyes. It was hard for her to focus.

Someone grabbed her wrists while another person cleaned the blood from her head and eyes. She forced her eyes open and wished she hadn't. She saw Father Jonathan holding Stephanie back. Stephanie wanted to finish the job she had started. Jenny was happy to see the large priest holding Stephanie about two feet off the ground. Jenny felt zip ties being placed on her wrists. She could see someone tending to me. I was woozy but I sat up.

Stephanie screamed. "Let me at that bitch. Give me five minutes and come back."

Father Jonathan put her on the ground and patted her on the head. He still had a good hold on her. "Stephanie, you saved ZZ's life. I know you want revenge but this, "bitch," may be able to help us."

Azzie wanted to call an ambulance for me, but my head was clearing and I declined. Joe wanted to call the police, but I thought that ought to wait.

Joe asked me. "ZZ this was close, what do you want to do?"

"For now, let's take her home with us. We need some time to figure out our next moves."

Joe advised me. "We can't take her against her will. That would be kidnapping."

I shot back. "It might be in her best interest to come with us."

Jenny was defiant. "Why would that be?"

I offered, "We might be able to work something out."

"There isn't much to work out. We came here to have sex and you wanted to shoot up first."

"That's not what went down."

"You can't prove that," Jenny screamed

Stephanie stood and approached Jenny. Father Jonathan held one of Stephanie's arms to assure himself that she would not strike Jenny. Stephanie brushed him off.

"I am fine, I just want to show her a great video."

She proceeded to show Jenny a video of her and I that started right after our arrival at the lake. It was embarrassing to watch the sex act on my sister's phone but the video did show Jenny adding pills to my wine glass. It also clearly showed that I had passed out when Jenny pulled out the fentanyl and applied the tourniquet.

Joe added, "That video plus an analysis of the strength of the dope you were about to give him should be conclusive proof of attempted murder. You can come with us voluntarily, or we will hold you here until the police arrive. Your call."

Jenny whispered, "I will listen to your offer."

We piled into our cars. Father Jonathan sat beside Jenny in the back seat in case she tried to flee. Joe drove. Azzie took me home in my truck after stopping to get me coffee. Stephanie worked her way to the other side of the lake and recovered her truck.

CHAPTER 53

Fired Up Farms
1915 August 15

Dad and Mom returned from the hospital when they got the call that I was ok. Mom warmed the remaining pizzas in the oven and waited for all to arrive.

I was still a little foggy, but I felt much better than I had at the lake. Mom glared at Jenny as she was escorted in the door by Father Jonathan. It was decided that Joe and I would interview Jenny. We took her into the den and closed the door.

I began. "Why? Why?"

Jenny cried and sobbed "I'm sorry, so sorry."

Joe wasn't buying it. "Save it for someone who believes your bullshit. Now ZZ, you can interrupt me, but here are the terms I propose. First Jenny, you tell us everything, and I mean everything, you know about your uncle, his hospital operations, and his racing operations. Second, you tell us what you know about his dealings with Adam Jurovich. Third, you tell us why you tried to off ZZ. Fourth, you tell us anything you know about the "accident" that Carl Zander did not cause, that killed Ken Harrow."

Jenny stopped crying and the negotiating ensued. "What's in this for me? My uncle will kill me if he finds out I gave you any information. Jail might be a safer alternative."

I spoke up. "Provided the information you give is good and truthful we will destroy the evidence of my attempted murder."

Joe added. "We can hide you until we get Deuce in police custody. It may take a few weeks but you will be safe. Were you supposed to call him when you had killed ZZ?"

Jenny shook her head. "No, he did not want me to have any contact. He said he would either hear it on the news or know that the body hadn't been discovered yet if ZZ didn't show at the track, Saturday. How do I know that you won't just take my information and then turn me into the police?"

I responded. "No guarantees, but you know me. You also know your uncle. Who would prefer to deal with?"

Jenny agreed. She began her confession by saying that the only thing she knew about Dad's wreck was that she switched tubes for his blood alcohol level. She was given a tube with a high blood alcohol level that she substituted for the one she drew.

Joe dug deeper. "Who asked you to do that?"

Jenny responded, "My Uncle, Thomas Hofecker."

Joe inquired. "Do you do everything your uncle tells you?"

Jenny nodded, "Pretty much."

Joe pressed the issue. "Why?"

Jenny asked, "How much do you know about the Jurovich case?"

"Everything that was in the paper. Is there something else we should know?"

Jenny relented. "I have very little recall of the evening."

I interrupted. "Isn't that convenient?"

Jenny continued. "Say what you want but here's all I know. Deuce told me that Jurovich was married and was going to dump me. I started drinking heavily. I called Aaron and convinced him to come over. I remember loading my gun and putting on the silencer before he arrived, and then I blacked out. The next thing I knew I woke up on the floor with my gun in my hand. Jurovich was lying next to me, dead. I looked up and Knuckles was standing over me. He told me that I killed Jurovich but if I listened to what he had to say I could get off. The next thing I remember was waking up in the hospital with a broken jaw, orbital fractures, and tons of other injuries. The police were there but before they could question me my attorney stopped them."

Joe inquired. "Did you have an attorney before that?"

Jenny laughed. "No, of course not. This guy was the best defense attorney that money could buy, and my uncle bought him."

I figured it out. "So that's why you owe him."

Jenny laughed again. "Partially. My attorney played up my severe facial injuries to the prosecutor. The pictures of my face were incredibly graphic. Two neighbors told police that they heard the sickening sounds of the beating I took. I had no previous record. The prosecutor had been elected on a platform of zero tolerance for domestic abuse. My attorney convinced him that I had been a victim and acted in self-defense. I was not charged with a crime."

Joe dug deeper. "Did your uncle know Jurovich?"

Jenny chronicled the events with Adam Jurovich. She met him and began an affair with him prior to her uncle coming to visit. So, Deuce did not instigate it. But once he found out what Adam did, he befriended him. They spent a lot of time together.

I wasn't connecting the dots just yet. "So, big damn deal. He paid for an attorney that got you off. It was nice of him, but it hardly gives him leverage to blackmail you."

Jenny agreed. "That's right. But shortly after I was free to leave Florida, he told me that he knew I was guilty of murder. He said he had clear evidence that I had not been injured before Aaron was killed. He said that with that evidence the prosecutor could reopen the case and file murder charges. The only defense I had was the self-defense claim and the evidence ruined that. He threatened to reveal it anytime he wanted me to do something."

I had to know. "Like kill me?"

Jenny bowed her head. "Exactly. He said that if I got you to disappear, he would give me the evidence. Therefore, I would be free of him for good. But before that he made me move to New Jersey and work in the ER so I could do his favors."

Joe pressed her, "Were you scheduled to work the night that Carl Zander had his wreck?"

Jenny shook her head no, "I was off that night, but they always called me in when blood alcohol levels were needed if I was in town."

That didn't make sense to me. "That's crazy. Anyone can draw a blood alcohol."

Jenny laughed, "But Deuce, as you call him, wanted me to do as many as possible. He concocted some story for the staff about a lawsuit we got because the blood alcohol paperwork and chain of evidence weren't properly done. It wasn't true but no one knew that.

"I still don't follow," I said.

Jenny smiled again. "ZZ, it's simple. Deuce had a nice thing going with doing favors for people. Of course, he would not know when someone in need of a favor might be arrested. So, I got called for most blood alcohols from 8 PM until 7 AM. Once I got there and found out who the patient was I called or texted Deuce. I would go ahead and draw the blood and wait for him to get back to me. If he could make a deal with the person or their attorney, he texted me to switch the tubes. I always had half a dozen tubes with blood alcohol levels under the legal limit. If he didn't know them or had no deal the originals were submitted. If I wasn't available, the charge person drew and processed the blood as usual. Deuce would only work with me."

I was putting the pieces together. "Tell me about drawing Dad's blood."

Jenny responded, "I got the samples and texted Deuce. He told me to substitute a 'hot tube', meaning one that was loaded with alcohol. I did it."

Joe had a question. "What was Carl's blood alcohol?"

Jenny answered, "I have no idea. I threw it out."

That cleared up a few questions that we all had. Dad had little recall, but no one saw him drink more than one drink. But for the plan to work Dad had to have a blood alcohol level that exceeded the legal limit. Deuce had Jenny take care of that.

That brought me to surmise, "If Dad's blood alcohol wasn't high then Ken Harrow's was probably under the legal limit too. Were you told to do anything about Ken?"

Jenny thought for a second, "The other victim was pronounced dead at the scene, so he was not brought into the ER. I only switched tubes in the ER."

That led to a discussion between Joe and I about how Ken's blood alcohol level at autopsy was found to be severely elevated. Jenny interrupted us.

"The coroner is old and drunk most of the time. He is also good friends with Knuckles. I know for a fact that Knuckles often goes to the morgue when the coroner comes in. He easily could have switched the samples for Ken's blood alcohol."

Things were starting to add up.

I had to know more. "Jenny, in addition to working full time you were on call almost 11 hours a day. I know Deuce was blackmailing you but that seems a bit much."

Jenny fessed up. "He paid me well. I got $1,000 for each switched tube. He paid me cash and made me deposit most of it so there was a record. I made close to $60,000 last year.

I was incredulous. "Sixty switched tubes?"

Jenny shook her head no. "Some of that money was for trial testimony."

I was getting a headache. "What trials? If you switched the tubes to a result below the legal limit the police would be hard pressed to bring charges."

Jenny laughed again. "ZZ, you are such a choir boy. Other than accidents we only drew blood alcohols on people who had been arrested for DUI. They had failed field sobriety tests and were brought to the ER after they had been arrested. Pretty hard to get a DUI conviction with a blood alcohol less than 0.08. But that would then open the door to false arrest suits. That's where Deuce made the big bucks. I got $5,000 each time I had to testify. Most of these 'wrongly accused' were prominent citizens. Most verdicts were for $200,000 or more."

Joe shook his head. "What a racket. He knew he could control you with the blackmail threat, but he also paid you well. Just another insurance policy for him. With you as part of the scheme, you were much less likely to rat him and Knuckles out. Clever. What else did he blackmail you to do?"

Jenny gave more details. "I was told to befriend ZZ when he started working in the ER. I was to find out as much as I could about his family and the farm. He was really interested in their farm. Other than that, he wanted me working the night shift in the ER. That was when most suspected drunk drivers were brought in."

I had to know if I was right in my suspicions. "Was Buster one of the ones that owed."

Jenny nodded. "You guessed right. He was shitfaced one night and hit an old lady in a crosswalk, who died. His blood alcohol was 0.248 but when the lab reported the sample I had substituted it was 0.064. He got off easy."

Jenny then listed a number of medical staff members, two board members, and a few prominent members of the community who "owed" Uncle Tom.

I was starting to feel sorry for her, but I wasn't letting on. "OK, what can you tell us about Supreme Medical and the racing operation?"

"Not much there. He never mentioned it to me. I had never been to the races before you took me. He did ask me to find out as much as I could about how Fired Up Farms operated though."

Joe asked, "What about the hospital?"

"Well, I can't help too much there either. He never talked to me about the hospital unless there was a blood alcohol level that I needed to substitute. I worked nights so I wasn't around for most hospital gossip."

I pressed her. "The hospital became profitable around the same time as the stable. Any thoughts on that?"

"No, I arrived about two years after they bought the hospital. When I got there, things were pretty austere. But over the last couple of years the salaries and staffing have really improved. Most employees saw a vast improvement. They always have some "quality initiative' going, but I can't explain any sudden profitability."

I wasn't done yet. "Anything strange things that you heard or that you noticed?"

"Uncle Tom thinks your farm is a gold mine."

"What did he mean by that?"

"I have no freaking clue, but he said it many

times. The second strange thing that everyone notices is that the administrative offices are split into two sections. One is the public portion. That's where we have staff meetings etc. But there is supposedly a large suite adjoining the public portion that no one has access to except Uncle Tom and Knuckles."

Joe inquired. "Any rumors as to the reason for the suite?"

"None that I have heard. But there is a rumor that either Uncle Tom, Knuckles, or both are in that office 24/7."

That piqued my interest. "Isn't that odd?"

Jenny agreed. "Very, I have no explanation."

We placed Jenny in a spare but spartan loft in the barn. She made no objections. She declined any food. I found her some scrubs to wear to bed.

She looked at me as I handed her the scrubs. "ZZ, when this is over, I want a chance to prove that you can trust me. I think we have a future."

"Jenny, I would love to lie to you like everyone else does, but I won't. We need your help, and we will allow you to get off from trying to kill me. But you and I are done for good."

Jenny sobbed.

Back in the living room Joe and I filled the group in on what Jenny had revealed. A long discussion ensued.

"Ok, Azzie the brilliant, piece the dots together" teased Joe.

"My theory (Azzie said as she looked around the room) is this. Genny's meeting Jurovich was a fluke. Deuce happened to get to Florida and Genny told him about Jurovich, and what he did. Deuce knew the implications of CIC and figured that Jurovich could rig the computer system for CIC. Deuce befriended Jurovich through Jenny. He then confronted him with the fact that Deuce knew he was married, and Deuce would tell Jurovich's wife. A deal was struck and somehow Deuce was able to access or defeat the CIC security. Jenny was told about Jurovich being married knowing that she would react violently. Hopefully, she would kill Jurovich to cover up the secret deal. Boom boom boom, as Joe would say, it all worked out. Markovich set up the scene and gathered evidence that would implicate Jenny. Jurovich was dead and whatever Deuce could do to defeat CIC was born. Jenny owes Uncle Tom forever."

Joe nodded. "Plus, a murder investigation would likely have uncovered the depth of the relationship between Deuce and Jurovich. Getting the DA to not bring charges ended any further investigation. Pretty clean."

Dad commented, "Well, if they had the ability to defeat blood testing it could explain their sudden rise to the top in harness racing."

I felt I needed to add. "But we don't know that for sure, and the only for sure thing is that we can't prove anything."

Azzie blurted. "What we need is very likely in that hidden office in the hospital."

No one initially said a word, but one by one they agreed. The secret behind Supreme Medical and the key to the success of Supreme Stables probably resided in that office.

CHAPTER 54

Fired Up Farms
0700 August 16

At 3 AM we concluded our discussion with a recess until 7 AM. Four hours sleep was better than none but 7 AM arrived too early for everyone. Mom and Stephanie took off for the track. Joe took Jenny some breakfast and asked her to remain in her room. She agreed. Dad joined the group.

After breakfast the Dying Was Easy group plus my dad met. We held hands and prayed and hugged. We knew that most of us should have been dead. Joe, Azzie and Father Jonathan in the apartment, and me with Jenny. We thanked God again and then we looked at each other. With death out of the way to stop us, who could? And the answer was no one. We were fired up and no one gave a shit.

Father Jonathan led off. "We have to get in that office. There must be records of horse drugging that they don't want anyone to see."

Azzie added "I would bet that the evidence against Jenny is hidden there too."

Joe joined in "Getting into that office will not be easy."

I wondered how he came to that conclusion. "How do you know that?"

Joe smirked. "While you kids were sleeping, I got a friend with connections downtown to share with me some drawings of that office. For fire safety and disaster situations the hospital is required to keep current drawings on file."

Azzie was sympathetic. "No wonder you look so tired."

Joe smiled, "We can catch up on our sleep together when this is done."

Azzie had a grin on her face. Say no more.

Joe continued "That second office is a fortress. No hospital has or needs the security measures they have employed. They are hiding something big, and they are hiding it there. I think you all are right."

I tried to make a joke. "Ok, we break into the office. Pretty easy."

Joe scoffed. "If we somehow managed to gain entry we would most likely face an armed Deuce and/or Knuckles. But fear not. It is more likely that their security systems would give them a heads up, so they would call the police."

Father Jonathan woke up. "Then we have to get both of them out of there."

Azzie interjected "Jenny, and Joe's security friends from the hospital, claim that there is ALWAYS one of them there."

Dad spoke up for the first time. "Maybe there is way to get both of them out of there."

I was anxious to hear what Dad had to say. "Do tell, do tell!"

Dad went on to explain some history of Miracle Mile Racetrack. It was always known as an outlier in harness racing. It had some of the best races and some odd traditions. One tradition was "blue papering." Blue papering could only occur during Miracle Week, now known as Miracle Millions Week.

Dad detailed that "blue papering" started in the 50's. Apparently, some of the old gomers liked to race their horses for the owner's papers, the way kids raced cars for the pink slip. Harness papers at the time were blue, and hence the term "blue papering." The term was eventually shortened to "papering."

The other thing was that the track operators wanted as many horse owners at the track as possible when their horses raced. It was kind of like a country club thing. If they were there, they spent more and bet more.

There were a lot of rules about what you had to say, and when you had to say it. But if you did the right things you "papered" the horse that you wanted. That meant that if your horse beat their horse in that race, you got their horse after the race. You owned it. But if the "papered" horse beat yours, you lost your horse to them.

The owners of the "papered" horse had options provided more than 50% of the owners of the horse were at the track an hour before the race in question. For the privilege of scratching and not losing their horse, they had to pay the "paperers" an amount equal to the purse of the race that they had entered.

If more than 50% of the owners were not present in the required time frame the owners had to pay ten times the amount of the purse not to lose their horse. If no owners were there, the horse had to race.

Father Jonathan was confused. "That's interesting but how does that help our cause?"

Dad laid out the facts. "In the fourth race tonight, we have Fired Up Rio entered. Supremes have Supreme Jackpot. From what I have heard they think he will be a monster racehorse. It might be close, but I believe that if it comes down to it Rio can beat that horse. There are only two principal owners of Supreme Stables, Deuce Hofecker, (as ZZ would say), and Knuckles Markovich. If we "paper" that horse, I can pretty much guarantee that both of them will show up."

Azzie was intrigued "Why is that? How can you be sure?"

Dad responded. "I can't be positive but here's the numbers. The purse for the race is $100,000. If both owners show up, they can "save" their horse for $100,000. If only one is there they have to put up $1,000,000 to "save" their horse. The way they talk about this horse I know they will show up. They think he is worth a million or more. They won't chance losing him."

I was a little worried. "If they put up the money, fine. If they elect to race, we could lose Rio."

Dad wasted no time responding. "Not if you drive her the way I tell you! Just kidding ZZ. Yeah, we could lose her but if we don't get into the office and solve the riddles, it doesn't much matter does it? We lose everything next week if we don't turn things around."

Joe brought up a good point. "Let's assume for a second that Carl is right. We still have to get in that office. The more I study the plans, the harder this looks. You can forget about entering from the hallway. The doors and security systems they have on the door from there are out of this world. Tighter than bank vaults."

Azzie asked. "But don't they have to have two routes of egress in case of fire?"

Joe's face lit up. "Very good, sweet cheeks. You DO listen to the stuff I babble. Yes, they have to have a second route of exit. But that route is tied into the fire alarm system, and only opens in the event of an alarm."

The discussion continued about setting off the alarm. Numerous other ideas were floated for consideration. Joe listened, but his face and mind were buried in the plans. Then I heard some of the sweetest words on the planet.

"Boom, boom, boom" bellowed Joe. "We don't have to use the doors to enter. There is a cold air return duct that serves the office. Another part of that duct connects to one that serves the ante room for the morgue. If we can get someone into the morgue, they can get into the duct and work their way to the office."

I liked what I heard but I was still skeptical. "Even if they get into the office aren't there security systems that need to be defeated?"

Joe nodded in agreement. "Right you are. But from what I can tell the office systems are not on the life safety branch."

Dad pleaded. "Speak English, I'm a dumb horse trainer."

Joe obliged. "Hospitals are required to have backup generators. Obviously, they can't have the power go out in critical areas. Plus, heating, cooling and ventilation are very important in operating rooms and other areas. So, Medicare and other payers require backup generator(s). Long story short, the generators can't replace all electricity.

So, the hospital has to prioritize what is on, or not on, what is called the life safety branch. The life safety branch is powered by the generators. Anything on it gets power from a generator if the main power supply is interrupted. Anything not on it is off until the main power supply is restored. Getting back to how this affects our plan. All of the locks and cameras that have to do with the door that enters from the hallway are on the life safety branch. However, the security cameras and motion detectors in the secret office are not on the life safety branch."

I popped the obvious question. "What do you propose?"

Joe was ready. "We take out the main transformer serving the hospital. That will eliminate the security features inside the office."

That worried me. "Won't some patients die, or be severely affected?"

Joe reassured me "No big boy, relax. The generators provide enough power to more than meet the needs of the patients."

I needed to know more. "If we disable a transformer, how long does it take for NJ Electric to replace it?"

Joe anticipated the question. "They are required to fix a transformer serving a hospital within two hours.

Azzie stood. "To recap, we need to get into that office. To do that we need the office to be empty. "Papering" has been proposed as a remedy for that issue. We then plan to disable the main transformer to the hospital to deactivate the security measures inside the office. Because of the security measures outside the office, we need to access the office via an air duct that also serves the morgue."

Joe concurred. "That sums it up. I just hope I don't get my fat ass stuck in that duct."

Azzie protested. "Maybe my skinny ass will fit better!"

Joe shook his head. "I can't let you do that."

Azzie wasted no time. "Excuse me, you don't tell me what to do."

A long discussion ensued. Azzie got her way. Joe had to monitor the entire hospital situation, and there was a strong likelihood he would not fit. Azzie would try to enter the office when given the signal by Joe. Carl left to get to the track to enter the horses for the Miracle Millions races. He had to enter before 9am and it was 8:15. I stayed behind to help figure out how to get Azzie into the morgue.

CHAPTER 55

Security Gatehouse
Supreme Medical Center
1730 August 16

"What do you have?" the security officer asked the ambulance driver.

"30 year-old female, DOA from an auto accident on route 58." replied Amos.

"I didn't hear anything about that on the radio."

"Not surprising. This victim hit one of the cell towers that also held the EMS repeater for that sector. We had to use our backup phones to communicate. They are working on a temporary fix that should be up any time." Amos added with authority.

"Will the coroner be coming?" asked the security guard.

"I doubt it, his deputy was at the scene. We were asked to bring her here until the family makes arrangements. They were informed a short time ago."

"Ok, what is the name of the deceased?"

"Belinda Hightower."

"Put her in bin seven. Here's the keycard for the morgue. Bring it back to me when you are done."

Amos replied, "No problem." As he drove off, he said to the victim. "You better get under that sheet and have your blankets ready. We have to park outside and go down a corridor. Try to breathe as shallowly as possible. People really hate to see the sheets from a corpse moving up and down."

Azzie responded from under the sheets. "You got it. Now, once I am in the cooler, will I be able to get out?"

Amos gave her his final instructions. "I am going to put tape over the latch on the door to the bin we put you in. The door will close but not lock. Cover up, it will be cold. When Joe gives you the signal, come out and enter the duct and do your work. When you are finished, come back down the duct and get in the same bin. Father Jonathan will impersonate a funeral director and take you out on a gurney."

Azzie had to ask. "Do I really have to stay in the bin? Can't I just sit and wait in a chair or something?"

"Unfortunately, no. Between the hospital, the nearby nursing home, and EMS the morgue gets a fair amount of traffic. You cannot afford to be discovered."

When he had completed his task Amos dropped the key card back at the gate. He took the ambulance back to its station to finish the "oil change" he had supposedly performed.

An old man slowly approached the guard gate. His gait was unsteady.

"I was told your deputy cleared the stiff the ambulance crew just brought" said the security guard.

"What stiff?" mumbled the disheveled and obviously tanked coroner.

The security guard just shook his head and handed the sign-in sheet to the coroner. He couldn't help but think. "It's a good thing that old prick lives close enough to walk. If he was driving I would have to call the state police. Almost every Saturday he comes around to do paperwork. Every time he is dead drunk. How much could he get done? Oh well, what the hell do I care? Just another two hours and its Miller time for me."

Azzie propped the door to her bin open a little to let in some warmer air. Even with the blankets it was cold. She nearly wet herself when the door to the morgue suddenly opened. She very slowly and carefully positioned the bin door ajar just enough to see what was going on.

She didn't recognize the old guy. He was staggering and muttering. He wandered over to bin one. He opened the door and pulled out the drawer. He uncovered an elderly female patient and proceeded to drop his pants and climb up on the gurney. It was all Azzie could do not to vomit. She watched in horror as the old pervert tried to separate the deceased lady's legs. After a number of attempts he swore and climbed off the drawer. He closed bin one as he consulted a sheet of paper. She pulled her door shut without making a sound. Joe was never going to believe this.

Her shivering was interrupted when the door to her bin suddenly opened. The drawer that she was resting on slowly was pulled into the room. She peaked out from under the covers and saw that the old guy still had his pants down. That was bad, but even worse was the fact that he had half an erection. Azzie threw the sheets and blankets off and screamed. The coroner grabbed his chest and fell over backwards.

Azzie thought about checking for a pulse and doing CPR but in the end, she decided against it. After ten minutes passed, she checked for a pulse and found none. She dragged his body over near bin one and opened the door. She pulled out the drawer and uncovered the corpse. She placed the dead coroner face up on the floor. When he was found, there would be little doubt as to what that sick prick had been doing.

CHAPTER 56

Miracle Mile Racetrack and Casino

1800 August 16

"Ladies and gentlemen, may I have your attention" track announcer Gabe Vatter said after the national anthem had been completed. "Carl Zander has an announcement, Carl."

"Thank you, Gabe." Dad read from the script. The wording had to be exact. "Hear ye, hear ye, all racing fans present. Fired Up Farms of Krenshaw NJ hereby notifies Supreme Stables of Krenshaw NJ that their horse 'Supreme Jackpot' is hereby papered by Fired Up Rio in tonight's fourth race."

Gabe responded when Dad finished. "I have no idea what just happened here, but I will get you an explanation."

PC was camped out in the owner's clubhouse. He had $200,000 that he needed to turn into much more. *I better have a hot night.* PC picked his seat at the table to give him the best view of Deuce. Deuce was two tables away sipping a scotch and reading his program. One of the judges that PC recognized went over and said something to Deuce, and Deuce exploded like a volcano.

"What the fuck do you mean? Papered? Bullshit, this can't be." PC couldn't hear the judge but Deuce's face was violet and his eyes were bulging. When the judge finished, Deuce placed a phone call. He was still pretty much screaming, but PC couldn't make out much of what he said. The track announcer was explaining to the crowd what papering was, and the PA system was drowning out Deuce.

"Get your ass over here," Deuce yelled into the phone.

"Yo, Tom, you know I can't. I am waiting for a call on a big contract," Markovich replied.

"Fuck that, put the machine on. You have to get here in the next thirty minutes, or we could lose Jackpot. "

"How, why?"

"No time to explain. Get here and make it soon."

PC texted the group. "Deuce going nuts, screaming into his phone. Could not hear conversation but suspect Knuckles will be running out the office soon."

Father Jonathan had the hearse parked so he had a good view of the exit to the executive parking lot. Sure enough, Knuckles beat feet to his car and burned rubber out of the lot. Father Jonathan texted the group. "Tweedle Dee is off to join Tweedle Dum."

Joe texted Azzie. "Be ready. T minus ten seconds."

Joe pushed the button on the actuator. A small explosion occurred on top of NJ Electric generator 16-75-8988. All the buildings in a two-block radius of the hospital went dark. Eight seconds later some lights came back on at the hospital. Joe was relieved that the generator had started and that the transfer switches had worked properly.

Azzie turned on the pen light. She put a chair against the wall under the vent. The two screws securing the vent were easily removed. She carefully placed the vent on the floor and stood on the chair to hoist herself into the duct.

Father Jonathan left the hearse and took up his post in the hospital basement. From inside a janitor's closet, he had an excellent view of the door to the morgue. Now would be an inopportune time for anyone to enter the morgue. He had no idea what he was going to do to thwart it, but to be sure, no one was getting in there.

After entering the duct Azzie crawled along briskly until that duct intersected with another one at a ninety-degree angle. She turned right and continued her crawl until she saw a vent on the right. That vent was supposed to be on her left side. Something was wrong. She had silenced her phone, but still had it operational. She texted Joe.

"WTF? Vent on right. Isn't it supposed to be on left?"

Joe texted back "What can you see through the vent?"

"Looks like storage of some sort," came the reply.

"Ok, you turned the wrong way at the T. Go back. When you get to the T go straight another thirty feet."

When she did that, she arrived at a vent on her left. She peeked and was able to make out some office furniture. She carefully pushed the vent until the screw gave way on one side, then rotated the vent screen enough that she could fit through the opening. She then took the screw heads that Joe had given her and placed them in the screw openings on the vent, gluing them in position. Joe did not want the vent to have missing screws. When she left there was no way for her to replace them. Hence the fake screws. Upon leaving, she would tape the vent in place. From the room it would look normal.

Joe had been 90% certain that the alarms in the office would not be operational. But he had no idea about any cameras. Azzie was dressed in black with a black hood and black gloves. She located two cameras and went to work. Father Jonathan had given her an app that she used to interrogate the cameras. On both cameras she saw herself walking toward them. She backed up until the lights went out. At that point she used the app to reprogram the cameras to loop themselves every 15 minutes for the next hour. When anyone looked at the tape, they would see the lights go out and eventually come back on after an hour or so. But there would be no record of Azzie's presence. At least that was the theory.

She texted Joe "In, cameras edited, going to work."

PC texted the group "Tweedle Dee arrived at track, will keep you posted if he departs."

Azzie began at the desk nearest the vent. It was small, and luckily it was unlocked. She found nothing of any value, and nothing that could store any computer information. She saw some light around the bend. She slowly crept around the corner and there was a laptop on a large desk. It was on but was running on battery power. She examined it carefully and took pictures of it with her cell phone as Joe had told her to do. When she had finished that she hit one of the keys and the monitor came alive. The machine wanted her password. She typed "PASSWORD." The machine replied "Entry Denied." Then she tried "password". To her surprise she was in the system.

She had been instructed not to look around on the computer. Instead, she was to insert a device that would copy the hard drive. She connected the device and the screen told her the download would take thirty minutes. She texted Father Jonathan. He thought that was reasonable.

She had to pee badly, and her bladder nearly obliged her when the office phone rang. She counted five rings, then she heard an answering machine. "You have reached Confidential Solutions, please leave a message. This is a secure line."

The caller left a message as directed. "Hey guys, I thought one of you were always there. Ok, so maybe you are on the can or something. This is Repairman. My client has a problem that needs your help. His problem is on its way to Florida tonight. Expect report next week. 1000K now, 1000K for full-year coverage. I will wire deposit when you confirm. Seven, capital B, small z, One, Nine, capital T, capital V, 7, small r, small d, 4, capital M, Capital Z, capital G, 7, 7, small b, small b, 5, small k."

Azzie recorded the message on her phone. She still had about twenty-five minutes and she began to look around. There was not much in the desk. She looked in every closet and found nothing suspicious. She looked behind pictures for hidden safes and found none. Her sleuthing was interrupted by a beeping on the device she had attached to the computer. Shit, she thought as she read the message "Download Failure." She texted Father Jonathan.

He texted back. "Shut down device, and computer. Restart each separately. After you have signed back into the computer, connect and try again."

Azzie repeated that process and got a different message. 55 minutes to download. They didn't have that much time. She sent the information to Father Jonathan and within a minute she received his reply.

"There is a small keyboard on the device. Type in 'Shorten download' and hit enter."

She did and the device informed her that the download would be done in 35 minutes. She later learned from Father Jonathan that a shortened download only captured text. No pictures or video, hence it was much smaller and faster.

She looked at her watch. It was 1852. Their only hope was that Knuckles stayed and watched some races. There was nothing she could do about that now. She continued her search. The bookcase was impressive. But when she looked up at an angle, she noticed four books on the third shelf appeared different. She got a chair and reached up. She pressed on one of the books and a door opened. A door that was composed of the fake spines of the four books. The open door revealed a wall safe. She touched the handle of the safe and it opened. Lucky day! She reached in and pulled out a box filled with envelopes. Various people's names had been written on the front of the envelopes. There was no envelope for Jenny Rich. She consulted her phone for the name Jenny had used in Florida. Gennifer Poorman did have an envelope. Azzie put it her pocket. She considered taking all the envelopes but decided against it. One missing envelope might go unnoticed, an empty safe would be obvious.

Knuckles arrived in the clubhouse at 1855 and one of the judges was summoned. Knuckles wanted, and got, an explanation of Papering. From what PC could see there was some disagreement amongst the Supremes.

At 1900 we got our answer via the track announcer.

"Ladies and gentleman, please note that we have a late scratch in tonight's fourth race. Please scratch number six, Supreme Jackpot. This is a judge's scratch. Supreme Stables has elected to forfeit $100,000 to Fired Up Farms so as to not have to race him against Fired Up Rio for papers. Fired up Rio will race."

PC texted all. "Tweedle Dee leaving clubhouse and appears to be in a hurry. Be prepared for his ETA back at hospital by 1945."

Azzie thumbed her reply. "Not sure the download will be done."

Father Jonathan ordered. "When I give you the signal, remove the device. We will have to take what we can get. Make sure you shut down the computer and don't leave any prints."

CHAPTER 57

Private Administrative Office
Supreme Medical Center
1924 August 16

Azzie's phone vibrated again.

"Get moving" was the short text from Father Jonathan. She grabbed the device and popped it free of the computer. She shut the computer down and then restarted it, so it was the way she found it. She took seconds she did not have to replace the hairs exactly the way she found them. Her memory was helped by the pictures on her phone. When that task was finished, she hoisted herself into the vent. She carefully pulled and taped it back into place. Slowly she made her way back to the morgue. The coroner was still dead, face up on the floor, pants down and chubby intact. There was no sense jumping back in the bin. If anyone came in now, there would be no way for them to miss the coroner. She sat and waited for Father Jonathan.

Ten minutes later the door to the anteroom slowly opened. A large man dressed in a black suit pushed a stretcher into the room. He raised his eyebrows when he noticed the recently deceased necrophiliac on the floor.

Azzie whispered, "Long story, let's get out of here. I will fill you in later."

Azzie gave him a quick hug and jumped into the body bag as Father Jonathan zipped it up. He uneventfully pushed the stretcher to the hearse and loaded it in the back. A few minutes later the hearse exited the hospital grounds. Azzie climbed out of the bag and crawled into the front passenger's seat. As she did that the parking lot lights came back on. The generator must have been fixed.

I won the first two races. They were catch drives, but I still got my driving commission. $1250 for each race. PC also made about $25,000 scoring big on the daily double. I was much more relaxed for the 4th race than I had anticipated. I would have liked the challenge of racing for papers, but I wanted no part of losing Rio.

She raced her heart out and was still not breathing heavily at the end. I had let her wander out of the gate. I didn't want her thinking she had to go to the front every week. With Jackpot scratched I had the luxury of racing her from behind. I got away sixth. At the ⅜ pole I pulled her to the outside and she went wild. Her third quarter was 26.3 seconds, and she won by 8 lengths in 1:52.4. Not bad for a fourth start. Unfortunately for PC Rio was an odds-on favorite. He made a dismally small profit on the race.

Fired Up Alabama made up for it. She had made breaks in two previous starts. But that was when Dad was incarcerated. He changed her shoeing and gave me a lecture on trotter's shoes. I don't like being lectured to, but I have to admit that tonight she was a dream. She trotted easily to the front, and I never had to start her up. She won jogging and returned $24.60 to win. PC had blasted her to win and used her heavily on top in exactas, trifectas, and the pick 4. He pocketed $150,000 on this race. He knew how and when to send it in and send it he did!

Supreme Taco continued her dominance of the Preferred Fillies and Mares. Tonight, she took a new mark of 1:48.1, and did it with ease. But it was another dismal return for PC. She paid a whopping $2.20 for a $2.00 bet. But she was nice and tight for next week's Filly and Mare $1,000,000 race.

Fired Up Nuke had been a stellar two-year-old but was injured and unraced at three. His first four starts this year produced two wins but tonight he was up in class. He had the lead at the top of the stretch. In mid-stretch he got on one line pretty badly and tried to break. I had to gather him in, and we finished fifth.

I shook my head as I responded to my Dad's questions. "Don't know Dad, he just isn't right. I think that stifle is still giving him some trouble."

"Could be ZZ, we'll back off. He isn't good enough to win next week anyway."

"Dad, I think everything turned out OK tonight." Meaning at the hospital.

"Good my son, good."

Fired Up Runaway had been slowly coming around the past few weeks. He was regally bred but had been pretty common on the racetrack during his two-year old races. This year, he got sick in May, and lost a lot of time. However, he won his last two starts and was beginning to show his class. Tonight, he was sluggish at the gate but responded when I reefed his ass a good one. He got the top at the ¼ but BB pulled Supreme Stag Party. We had to park him out. I really wanted to get Runaway a breather to the half, but that didn't happen. BB tried to get away going to the ¾ pole but I was able to keep Runaway within a length. Dad had taken his blinds off this week. I don't know if it was the Army, or the site of Stag Party on his outside but Runaway hit another gear at the top of the lane. From there on he was game to the wire. Stag party took a bad step and finished third. That put Dash of Salt in second at 99 to 1. I couldn't wait to see how PC had played it. That exacta was worth $1267.00 for a $2 wager.

CHAPTER 58

Fired Up Farms
2330 August 16

We reconvened at the farm. Stephanie, Mom and Dad would join us when they got the horses put away. PC had made $350,000. Nice night's work. Joe, Azzie and Father Jonathan had opened a bottle of wine and I grabbed a glass. Azzie handed me the envelope marked Port Saint Lucie evidence. There was a single photograph in there. We passed it around. It showed a very dead Adam Vucovich lying face up on the floor. His face and groin were covered in blood. Beside him Jenny was lying face up. In her right hand was a gun with a silencer. She appeared to be asleep or dead.

Joe was the first to speak after all had a chance to examine it. "I can see why Deuce kept this. Pretty damning to Jenny's defense. Look at her face. There isn't a mark on it."

I interjected. "Pretty clear that she killed him, and it wasn't in self-defense!"

Father Jonathan countered. "That picture doesn't prove she killed him."

Joe agreed and added another dimension to the discussion. "With this picture we do know for certain that Jenny did not act in self-defense. But we don't know if she was the one who killed Vucovich. Who took the freakin' picture?"

My head was swimming. I just couldn't venture a guess at his question, but I wanted to know what he thought. "Please Joe, I get the feeling you have a theory to explain everything. I would love to hear it."

Everyone in the room agreed.

Joe began. "Jenny has little recall of the events. She did admit to loading her gun and attaching the silencer, so she had intent. Jenny was found with the murder weapon in her right hand, and testing confirmed that she had fired it. But we don't know for sure that she killed him. We only now know that someone beat the living shit out of her before or after Vucovich began to assume room temperature. Was it the person or persons who took the picture? A picture that her prick of an uncle held over her head for years to extort her cooperation.

"I submit that Jenny and Vucovich were somehow incapacitated. Deuce and or Knuckles, or persons in their employ, put the gun in Jenny's hand and fired two shots at Vucovich. They then laid Jenny on the ground and took the picture. They waited for Jenny to come to a little and inflicted the beating of her life on her. Her blood alcohol level was 0.425 when she arrived at the hospital. That plus a severe concussion kept her quiet until Deuce got word to her. He planted the self-defense story and got her the best legal talent money could buy. Jenny was so damn drunk that she had no recall except for the script Deuce had given her. Now no one would ever look Deuce's way. The case was closed. Jenny was indebted to him forever, and the picture was his insurance policy."

I shook my head in disbelief. "Joe, you are brilliant. But that leads to another question. What do we do with Jenny? She still may be a murderer, but we don't know for sure. Plus, let's not forget that she tried to kill me too."

Azzie stood. "I for one think Jenny is a victim here. I think it went down exactly as Joe surmised. We all know Deuce and Knuckles are more than capable of setting something like that up. It was clear that they used Jenny to do their bidding. I think we should do nothing with her now except protect her. We certainly don't want to turn her over to the police or allow Deuce to get his hands on her."

After a 3-1 vote of the Dying Was Easy gang, it was decided that Jenny would stay at the farm as a guest. She would be free to leave but strongly advised not to. I was the lone dissenting vote.

I looked at Father Jonathan. "Now that we got that out of the way, when are you going to start working on the computer information that Azzie purloined?"

Father sighed "On it already. It is downloading into my PC. From there we can make copies and divide things up. We should be able to start in 10-15 minutes."

Azzie spoke up. "Let me play the phone call." She punched away at her phone and the recording played. "Mean anything to anyone?"

Joe nodded. "Sounds like someone buying an insurance contract of some sort. Usually, 1000K means $1 million dollars. One million now, and one million for a full year's coverage. Pretty expensive insurance."

I asked. "Anyone make anything of the letters and numbers? Twenty digits."

Father replied "Means nothing to me. Maybe our computer information can shed some light."

It didn't take long. Father gave Joe, Azzie, and I each a copy of the hard drive that Azzie had lifted. There were hundreds of files under three main sections: horses, athletes, and favors owed. I took horses. Joe took athletes. Azzie tackled favors owed.

Azzie had a question. "Little John, how much information do you think we are missing because I had to stop the download early?"

Father Jonathan smiled. "Actually, we got lucky. The only information we did not capture was from the horse's section. We got some but not all of that. However, we got 100% of the athletes and favors owed data."

The group was happy to hear that and immediately went back to work. No one said anything for about fifteen minutes and then a chorus of "holy shits" erupted.

Dad, Stephanie and Mom entered as the proclamations began.

Dad asked. "Father, are you having a GI disturbance?"

Father Jonathan answered. "I think I can use a change, if you know what I mean."

Azzie shook her head. "This is fucking incredible."

Stephanie corrected her. "Ah, Ms. Huggins, would you care to restate that?"

Azzie blew her off. "Some other time Stephanie, the f word is the only one I can use to describe what I think I saw."

Father Jonathan concurred. "Me too!"

I joined in. "No other word will do."

Dad couldn't wait to hear it all. "OK guys, spill your guts."

Azzie gave an abbreviated version of her night.

Stephanie didn't understand. "What was the coroner doing?"

I changed the subject. "I'll explain later Steph, but he is (was) one sick dude."

Joe and Father Jonathan filled in the details of the evening and gave a sanitized version of what we saw on the picture. Azzie played the phone call.

Stephanie shocked everyone. "That sounds like a CIC number."

Azzie was intrigued. "It does? How do you know about CIC?"

"When Dad went away, it became my job to register the horses with CIC and get their number. It's a twenty-digit thing, capital, and small letters, and numbers all mixed up."

Father Jonathan inquired. "How do you get this number?"

Stephanie quickly responded. "They have a website. You have to enter all kinds of information about the horse including chip numbers. Once they verify the stuff, they issue you a number. That is added to the electronic eligibility papers. The tracks enter it when that horse is required to have any testing."

I pondered that information and then asked. "What does everyone think of the call?"

Carl quickly answered. "Clearly someone wanting to buy something illegal."

Joe laughed. "And I think I know what that was."

All ears were on Joe. "My section was athletes. There are hundreds of names of famous athletes in there. With each name there is a date of acceptance, how much was paid up front, and how much was paid for future protection. It appears that college, professional and Olympic athletes were buying. I think they were buying freedom."

Mom didn't understand. "Freedom from what?"

Joe quickly responded. "Freedom from detection of the use of performance enhancing drugs. PEDS for short."

I jumped in. "In the horse's section, I have lists of horse's names, and dates they were added, or deleted, from the system. Based upon Joe's report I would guess that these are the dates the horses were added, or deleted from, the ability for CIC to detect PEDS. Just as Jenny told us. Deuce got Vucovich to give him a way to have CIC report negatives for selected horses and clients."

Azzie added. "Deuce and Knuckles have a number of business lines. The first is that they can take care of athletes that need to use some banned substances or are caught using them. The second is that they can sanitize any horse they want to be immune from testing."

Father concurred. "We still have to confirm this, but that is how it appears at this point."

Azzie continued. "The third line of business was favors. And just as Jenny said, here are a list of prominent medical staff members, board members, and community leaders that may have benefited from Jenny switching a good blood alcohol tube for a bad one."

I had to ask. "Do we know anyone on the list?"

Azzie laughed. "Fancy that, we do. Buster, and a number of medical staff members, and guess who else?"

I couldn't wait for the answer. "I don't know."

Azzie shrieked. "Not Too Juicy Lucy!!! Do you want a trifecta????"

I was all ears, and they were separated by a huge grin.

Azzie continued. "Old Lady Bradshaw!"

I shook my head. "Damn, I should have guessed her. That old battle ax sure did all she could to screw me. I would never have guessed Not Too Juicy Lucy."

Joe was laughing uncontrollably. "That old spinster could probably drink your ass under the table."

Mom looked at her watch. "How about a nightcap, and we all hit the hay. Sunrise is about five hours from now, and I am looking forward to a sunrise mass."

Father Jonathan slapped his forehead. "Whoops I forgot, but we did promise the kids."

We skipped the nightcaps and hit the sheets.

CHAPTER 59

Fired Up Farms
0600 August 17

The morning air was refreshing but not cold. The Army and their therapists were ecstatic. We held small candles as the service began. One of the therapists played a hymn on the portable organ that we carried from the school to the start line of the training track. That's where the service was conducted. Father Jonathan held everyone spellbound with one of his greatest sermons yet.

He talked in terms that the kids could understand. He explained the importance of a fresh start. That we all are sinners. And just like a horse that runs a bad race, we often get many chances to make a fresh start. It's how we take advantage of the opportunities that we are given that makes the difference. There was a difference between learning from past mistakes and allowing past mistakes to define and overtake you.

It was pitch black when he started. Even though he kept his sermons short when the kids were involved, the sun had risen by the time he finished. In the paddock near the start line Always Hope stood silently with her suckling colt at her side. When Father Jonathan finished, she turned and ran into the field kicking and whinnying. She was followed by her colt, who tried to do much the same. The kids went wild. Father Jonathan shook his head but out of the corner of his eye he noticed someone watching him from the barn loft. It was Jenny, and she was on her knees.

Breakfast with the kids was sheer bedlam but it was fun. After the kids were fed and the school cafeteria cleaned, we adjourned to the house. We all had jobs to finish. I suggested a report out at noon.

Father Jonathan went first. "Our suspicions were correct. Deuce and Knuckles had been given a way into the CIC system. It took a while, but I found a scanned document in what appears to be Deuce's handwriting that details the system. It ties in with the 20-digit numbers Stephanie alluded to. Vuckovich built a door into the registration system. That was brilliant. Most people would look at the mainframe that spit out the results for evidence that people were hacking . People are adding information into the registration system all the time. So, there was much less chance of anyone noticing."

I was intrigued. "How do they get from doctoring the registration to having the mainframe spit out bogus negative results?"

Father was flustered. "Damn it ZZ, can I finish?" He paused. "Sorry everyone, I'm very tired but I've got to get my language back under control. I will be cleaning the bishop's floors with my toothbrush if I am not careful. And ZZ my friend, I will be glad to answer all questions when I am done."

I stood and put my arm around him. "Love ya, man."

Father grinned. "You too, ya goof. Now back to business. The scanned document laid it all out. Deuce or Knuckles had to have the original CIC number for the horse or athlete that they wished to test negative. Then they had to access the registration system at exactly 2 AM EST."

Stephanie raised her hand.

Father acknowledged her kindly. If it was me, he might have exploded. "Yes, my dear?"

Stephanie apologized. "Sorry to interrupt, but I know the system is down around 2 AM. Once or twice, I tried accessing it during that time and I got a damn error message."

Father agreed. "Right you are. That is how Vuckovich set this up. From 2-2:15 AM daily the registration system takes itself offline to perform diagnostics and routine self-maintenance. Anyone attempting access during that time would get an error message. The error message has the CIC logo at the bottom left of the page. If you happen to click the logo nothing happens. But if you click the logo and type in GENNY, all caps, within five seconds, it takes you to a different screen."

There wasn't a sound in the room.

He continued. "On that screen there are two rows of twenty- digit blocks, one on top of the other. They enter the existing CIC number in the top and in the bottom, they enter the 'recognized as' number."

Dad protested. "I am getting lost."

Father begged. "Stick with me. This may sound complex but when I am done you will see it is not. The mainframe did have one little quirk built into it. It had a secret code that permitted it to be told to read one number and recognize it as a second number instead. The mainframe had also been programmed that when certain letters, or numbers appeared in certain digits that the computer would generate negative reports for all samples submitted.

Dad still was confused. "Maybe I drank too much booze in my younger days, but I still don't get it."

Father was patient. "Let me make it simple. Say we used three-digit numbers instead of twenty. They needed twenty to allow them to register tons of athletes and horses but say they only needed three. And what if you programmed the computer that anytime the second character was a small g, 'g,' that the computer would enter a negative result?

"So, if the number was 46F, or 7Bw, or 157 the computer would result exactly what was found. But if the computer came across say 4gH, or gg6 the small g in the second character spot would make the computer spit out a negative result regardless of what was actually found.

"So, armed with the original, permanent registration number, Deuce or Knuckles could access the registration computer between 2-2:15 daily to create what they called 'recognized as' numbers. The computer still reported the results to the original number but the 'recognized as' number made the results all negative.

"When a client's subscription ran out, or if they sold, or had a horse claimed, Deuce and Knuckles went back into the system and removed the 'recognized as' numbers. Normal testing results would again be reported."

Joe was amazed. "Boom, boom, boom, they owned the system that supposedly couldn't be hacked. Actually, they weren't hacking it, they just used a feature that no one had access too. That sucked, but it was a brilliant suck."

Dad now understood. "Father, can you also get into the system?"

Father responded, "Now I can, why?"

Dad answered. "If you were to access the system tonight, would you be able to remove the fake numbers so the testing would again be legit?"

Father shook his head up and down. "I believe so."

I jumped in. "Let's shut the bastards down tonight. There should be plenty of samples from horses the Supremes raced this week on their way to, or in Florida by now. We know that most of them will be positive. Once a bunch of their horse's positives are reported to the track stewards, they will shut them down. Supremes will either not be able to race or will have to race their horses without PEDS. Either way we clean up during Millions Week."

Dad was concerned with that approach. "Can you imagine the impact on horse racing when this info hits? They could cancel or postpone Millions Week. We can't afford that."

I knew he was right. "They would have to shut things down until they got a grip on it. No one would wager a dime there until they knew that the races were honest, and horses were not taking PEDS."

Dad agreed. "But if Father deactivates the RA numbers after Millions Week we can have it all. Say we win four races on Millions Night and ten other races during the Millions Week. We still come up short of the cash we need. But in a few days after the race the shit will hit the fan. All the Supreme horses will have positives and they will have to forfeit any purse money. If all we do is win or finish second to them, we will eventually get the full purse money."

Mom had a rare question. "But if they win and appeal the positive finding, they could tie this up for months, couldn't they? They have the right to have the split samples examined. Then they can try to explain things away with excuses like they had contaminated feed etc."

Joe asked. "What's a split sample?"

I jumped in. "When samples are taken after a race they are split into two samples. In the event that the first sample tests positive the trainer involved can request that the split sample also be tested to verify the result. The split samples are usually kept for six months."

Dad then answered Mom's question. "For most of the year you are correct. But the rules of Millions Week are clear, and like Millions Week, they are a little different. Any positive requires an automatic, and immediate testing of the split. If the split confirms banned substances the trainer has five days to present an appeal. No extensions are permitted. The process is over in less than fifteen days after the race. If the Supremes have as many positives as I think, they will not succeed in appeals. They might be able to explain away one or two, but ten or more will be insurmountable.

Father grinned as he proclaimed. "At 2 AM, the Sunday morning after the Miracle Millions race, we change the course of racing history. What about the athletes?"

I had already been pondering that. "With only fifteen minutes to work each night there will be time constraints. For each horse we have to enter a 20-digit number and enter a new 20-digit number. We have to get all of the horses that race for Supremes during Millions Week 'clean' first. But it would be my vote that as time permits, after the horses are done, that you remove all of the RA numbers."

Azzie had been silent for a while. "Why remove any athletes? Let the FBI shut it down."

I shot back. "Because I don't totally trust the FBI. They sometimes appear to have political leanings, and this will cause a hullabaloo. I worry that the FBI leadership will bow to political pressure to suppress this. I spent some time looking over the client list. We are talking about every major professional sport in this country. That is big enough but add to that a majority of NCAA football and basketball teams also have players on the list. Throw in the Olympians and every senator and congressman will want to shut down any scandal affecting their constituents, and more importantly schools and teams supported by their big donors."

Joe made a great point. "We've got another problem folks. It's cut and dried with the horses. They raced and therefore we know the winners at least will be tested. The athletes are a different story. They are tested randomly. We have no guarantee that anyone whose number we deactivate will be tested soon."

I cringed. "Joe is exactly right. We can't count on current testing to expose the athletes. Once the positive horse samples come to light action could be taken to prevent discovery of the cheating athletes. But we know that CIC has six months-worth of split samples from the athletes. We have to encourage someone to analyze those."

Joe added. "If the FBI was inclined to do a cover-up, the best way would be to get custody of the splits before they were analyzed. If they made sure they tested negative there would only be positive tests in harness racing. The athletes would get off scot-free."

I thought out loud. "We all want every cheating athlete, corrupt trainer, profiteering owner, and unscrupulous agent brought to justice. How do we manage that?"

Azzie jumped to her feet. This was right in her wheelhouse. "First of all, we choose one media outlet to break the story. At the same time the story breaks we appeal to the governor of the state where the splits are kept. In this case, Florida. ZZ, Isn't your friend, our governor, good friends with the governor or Florida?"

"As a matter of fact, he is. And since Millions Week will occur in his state and the main perpetrators of PEDs cheating reside here, I am sure the governor will want to be out in front of this as it unfolds."

Azzie grinned. "Both governors could garner a lot of great publicity, and make sure the whole caper gets exposed. ZZ, when we are done here would you do the honors of contacting the governor?"

"My pleasure."

Azzie had it all coming into focus. "We ask both governor's help in securing the splits so the FBI alone cannot get them. Shortly after that we take to social media and release every name we have. We caution the public that anyone, or agency, that attempts to confiscate the splits might be part of a cover up."

Joe was amazed. "Two points. First, the FBI will eventually be able to get the splits. This is so widespread that the FBI is the most logical agency to take charge. Second, can we get in any trouble for releasing the names?"

Azzie jumped back into the discussion. "We can get Dan's advice about how to release the names without any trace to us. If we play our cards right, I think we can put pressure on the FBI to have the CIC personnel do the testing on the splits after the RA numbers are removed. With the help of the governors and some of my contacts in the media we should be able to gin up enough of an outcry to force the FBI to allow unbiased witnesses to view all handling of the splits. Coverups depend on dragging things out and suppressing evidence. The more facts that we can get out quickly can stop the coverup before it gets started."

There were no more questions on that subject. Azzie would first talk with Dan and then coordinate the leaks and social media posts that would make the shitstorm a reality. Another topic that hadn't been settled was what to do with the people on the favors owed list.

Joe was first up. "For now, nothing. But there are a ton of doctors and politicians on there. They need to be exposed."

Dad spoke up. "I agree. But that is probably best left for another day."

I concurred. "OK, this week we concentrate on racing and starting Saturday night Father Jonathan will start to deactivate numbers. Azzie, Joe, you guys have sacrificed a ton of time. We will need you here for next Saturday but if you need to leave this week to tend to business, I know we can handle things here."

Azzie was skeptical. "Are you sure? I am into the end."

Joe joined her. "Me too!"

I smiled. "You can coordinate the leaks and media response from your locations. You do not need to be here. See you next Saturday."

Father Jonathan interrupted me. "Just one last thing before we split up. What are we going to do with Jenny? She can't be forced to stay in the barn much longer."

I hadn't changed my mind. "She can rot out there for all I care."

Father rebuked me. "What part of love thy enemies don't you get?"

I had to admit. "I am a little weak in that area. You weren't drugged and nearly…." I stopped in mid-sentence. "Oh yes you were, and then you were dipped in shit. Have you forgiven them?"

Father was duly humbled. "Still working on it but I am making some progress. Jenny has expressed a number of things to me, including the fact that she gave us valuable information. We had promised to give her the evidence back."

I was scared to death. "Father, you didn't talk to her alone? She is a sociopath. She will allege you molested her and blackmail you with the bishop. You know how those investigations go. Guilty until proven guilty."

Father laughed. "ZZ, I know you are brilliant but the rest of us do have an occasional lucid thought. I spoke with Jenny at her request but I had a visual chaperone. They were out of earshot but had a video going of the interaction."

Stephanie spoke up. "I like taking videos of Jenny. Want to see it?"

This time I was the humble one. "Sorry Father, I should have known better. What do you suggest?"

He continued. "I suggest that Jenny be allowed to move into Azzie's room, and eat and interact with us. Of course, when we have team meetings or any discussion of sensitive information those will have to happen at the school."

I gave in. "She would be relatively safe here. Clearly Deuce has to know that she failed. He may be looking to take her out."

Dad added. "We need to beef up our security here too. Everyone needs to know the combination for the gun cabinets. The weapons need to be loaded. Deuce and Knuckles may send their goons here when they find out that the picture is missing. By now we have to assume that they tried to find it to repay Jenny for her failure."

Joe agreed. "Before we leave, I will check the surveillance equipment and alarms."

I asked the group. "Do we give the picture to Jenny?"

Father cautioned. "I wouldn't bring that up until she does. She is trying to sort out her options. But I would get it out of here to someplace safe. I only trust her to a point. Do you have a safety deposit box?"

Dad agreed to take the letter to the bank tomorrow. An hour later Azzie's helicopter landed and took off again in five minutes. Joe hitched a ride. I helped Mom change the sheets in Azzie's room. She was the first to speak.

"Zachary, I didn't want to argue with Father Jonathan, but I really don't trust Jenny."

"Well Mom, of course I don't either. But Father Jonathan said he would take total responsibility for her. That reminds me, I need to arrange for a female therapist from the school to come here when Father Jonathan meets with Jenny. We need to make sure that Jenny is never alone with him. No need to tempt her."

CHAPTER 60

Fired Up Farms
0530 August 18

5:30 came pretty early. The smell of bacon cooking and fresh hot coffee emanated from the kitchen. I was only half awake when I turned the corner, but I woke up when I saw Jenny laboring over a hot stove. She was the first to speak.

"Nothing gets a day started better than a hot breakfast! Can I get you some coffee?"

"I can get it. You have your hands full."

"I hope you like scrambled eggs, it's too hard to cook eggs to order for six people."

"I love them. Can you add a little sour cream to mine?"

"Ah, the Gordon Ramsey method." She grinned at me.

"Look ZZ, everyone will be down soon, so I need to make this quick. I meant it before when I asked your forgiveness. I promise you that I will cause no trouble here and that I will do my best to help you folks. I am still trying to figure out what I am going to do. I really appreciate being able to stay here while I get my head together."

I decided to expose the elephant in the room. "You know the picture isn't here. We've put it someplace safe."

"I guess I deserve that and much more. But as of now I have no interest in that evidence."

For some stupid reason I believed her.

Father Jonathan ducked his head just in time to miss the top of the doorway. The old farmers that built these places must have been vertically challenged. "What do I smell?"

Stephanie, Mom, and Dad arrived within seconds of each other and took their places at a beautifully set table. It was covered with a bright, clean tablecloth. Incredibly arranged flowers from Mom's flower garden sat in the center of the table. A bowl of freshly picked blackberries sat in front of each plate.

Mom was appreciative. "Jenny, this wasn't necessary. You must have been working for hours. But the table is beautiful and the food smells delicious."

Jenny quickly responded. "It's about time I pulled my share of work. I owe each of you a great debt. I hope over time you come to see that I mean that."

Father smiled. "Can we say a prayer to start this off? Seems like a good idea."

We prayed and ate. Stephanie had the oddest frown on her face when she sat down. But after she dove into her food that frown was gone. That little sweetheart ate two helping of eggs, five pieces of bacon and three slices of toast. Not that I was counting. OK, so I was. But the important point is that she completed breakfast without uttering one expletive. There was no belching or other gas passages. Azzie had to work on her table manners but all things in good time.

Jenny refilled coffee cups as she asked. "Mrs. Zander, can I use the washer and dryer today? I have washed these in the sink for the past few days but they need some better cleaning," she pointed to her clothes that were piled in the sink.

"Of course." Mom said. "The detergent is in the cabinet above the washer."

Stephanie surprised me. "Jenny, I can take you to the school later if you like. The kids are constantly growing out of things. Azzie buys them clothes all the time. I am sure they have some that might fit you." She must have really enjoyed her breakfast.

Jenny started to cry. "You people should hate me, I tried to kill ZZ. How can you even look at me, let alone treat me nice?"

Dad spoke first. "It's hard but we are trying to remember not to throw the first stone, if you know what I mean. Let's get through this week and see where that takes us."

I turned my attention to Father Jonathan. He looked very tired. "Father, what are you doing today? You need a rest."

"Well, that won't happen. I made an appointment to see the bishop this morning. I really want to do about anything else, but I have to return next week. I thought I would try to mitigate his anger."

Jenny volunteered. "Would you like me to come with you?"

Father spoke before he thought. "Hell no!"

Jenny looked absolutely hurt. Father went on to explain.

"I took a personal leave of absence over the vehement objection of the bishop. If I show up to plead my case with a beautiful blond bombshell on my arm, I don't see it helping me much. This is something I have to do on my own, but I appreciate the offer."

Jenny understood. Stephanic gathered our things to get to the track. Dad reminded everyone of the team meeting conference call at 6 PM where we would review our financial situation and our plans for Millions Week.

Jenny spoke up. "Would there be a problem if I spent some time with the school nurse today? I ran into her yesterday during a walk near the school. She promised to give me a tour and explain a little of what she does over there. I think she was planning on updating physicals and I thought I could give her a hand."

I thought that was great. "There shouldn't be a problem, just keep your phone off. Don't make any calls or make contact with anyone else. We won't feel you are totally safe until Deuce and Knuckles are behind bars. Myra will take good care of you. She's one of the best hires I ever made."

Mom started to clear the dishes when Jenny held up her hand in protest.

"Please, you all have enough to do. I would appreciate it if you would go about your business. I will clean up."

Jenny was pleased when Mom agreed.

"Stephanie, can I see you in the living room for a second?" Jenny asked.

Stephanie and Jenny were gone for less than a minute. They returned to the kitchen where Stephanie pulled her coat off the rack and stopped at the door. "What kind of tampooooons do you want, and what size do you take? Do you like have to measure yourself or something? I'm a pad girl."

Jenny's face turned red. Father Jonathan took his coffee cup and scurried into the den as the rest of us hurriedly made our way to the door. Stephanie looked at us like we were crazy.

CHAPTER 61

Private Administrative Office
Supreme Medical Center
0700 August 18

"Did you find that little bitch?" Deuce was pissed.

"Not yet." Knuckles was taken back by Deuce's tone, but he had become used to his outrages. "We WILL find her!"

"Do we have any idea what the fuck happened?"

"The last ping we got on her phone was 8 PM Friday at the lake. We found her scooter parked where she told us she was going to put it. So, she didn't leave on the scooter. Other than that, we found shit."

"And her apartment?"

"I had a guy there all weekend, and nada. Plus, no use of credit cards, no emails, no texts. She just vanished."

"Niece or no niece, I've had it with her. I am going to send the picture to the prosecutor in Port Saint Lucie. You are pretty sure they will file murder charges?"

"Before you do that let's try to figure out how much Jenny knows and can prove. She will bargain her ass off to try to stay out of jail."

"When it comes to the murder, she will of course implicate you in telling her that Vuckovich was married. She may claim that you sanitized the scene and beat her."

"Did she ever see the picture?"

"No."

"Ok, so she has squat. Yes, I told her about him being married and I came over to console her after the incident. Did I disturb evidence? I might have. I'm not a cop. I am a friend of her uncle. I don't know how to act at a crime scene. As to beating her up, she was so drunk I am sure she knows nothing."

Deuce was still concerned. "She will tell them that I held the picture over her head and made her switch the blood alcohol tubes in the ER. She might even tell them that I told her to kill that Zander asshole."

Knuckles shook his head. "She can tell them I have butterflies shooting out my ass too, but she can't prove anything. Did you mention a picture specifically?"

"No, all I ever told her was that I had evidence that might cause the prosecutors to reopen her case."

"Good. She won't know for sure what to look for."

Deuce continued his interrogation. "What about the blood alcohols we had fixed for favors?"

"What about them?"

"She will, of course, tell the police about that."

"So?" Knuckles remained unfazed.

"But they will investigate."

"I can just hear it now. 'Councilman Driggs, did you have a DUI that Thomas Hofecker help you conceal?' asks the dumb dick policeman."

"'Of course, take me to jail and ruin my political career. I did it,' said Councilman Driggs." Knuckles laughed at his own sarcastic story.

"OK smart ass, none of the people who we did favors for will back up her story. It's not in their best interest."

Knuckles was happy that Deuce was seeing things his way. "You best get the word out to them that they may get a visit from the cops. Better for them to be prepared. But other than that, I vote we send that picture."

"You are sure it can't be traced to us?"

"We can make it look like it came from someone friendly to Vucovich's wife, like a private detective. They could not rule out a nosey neighbor peeping tom. They really don't need to prove the source if the picture is legit."

"Let me get it." Deuce walked over to the bookcase and opened the secret door. "What the fuck, what the fuck! The god damn picture is gone."

Knuckles was on his feet in an instant. "Gone? Can't be. Misplaced maybe, but not gone."

Deuce was livid. "Misplaced my ass, you twit. I put it in the safe a few years ago. I also keep our favors owed documents in there. Because of the security here I rarely lock it. It takes too long to enter the combination."

"That's brilliant!" Knuckles said in a very condescending tone.

"Fuck you too. Anyway, it's not in there."

"Any idea when it could have disappeared?'

"Absolutely none, I access that safe a couple times a week. I never thought I had to check to see if her envelope was there."

"What about last Saturday? You made me go to the track."

"Wasn't that the night of the power outage?"

"Yep, and you know how I hate coincidences." Knuckles was grim.

"Pull all tapes we have from the hallway, and here. Make sure we are not missing anything from the CIC operation. Do an inventory on the favors done folder."

"Yes sir." Knuckles agreed as he began his assigned duties. He really hated it when Deuce treated him like a lackey.

CHAPTER 62

Barn 7

Miracle Mile Racetrack and Casino

0700 August 18

The morning at the barn started like all others. Lots of stalls to clean, water buckets to fill, and manure to be pushed up the steep ramp to the collection bin. The pace was relaxed because we only had two horses to train today. Most others were just jogging. Stephanie finished her stalls first and started to get Rio ready to jog when she let out a scream.

"ZZ, she fucking lame, fucking lame!" Stephanie's speech had improved remarkably. But when she was excited, she mostly swore and left out some prepositions and other key grammatical components.

I ran to the hallway in front of the stall. Stephanie was in a complete meltdown. I took her lead (Rio's, not Stephanie's, although Stephanie needed one too) and I walked her down the hallway. She was dead lame and really favoring her front right leg. Just then Dad and Mom arrived in response to the 911 shriek from Stephanie.

We put Rio back in her stall in crossties. Dad looked like he had aged twenty years since breakfast. He had decided that Rio was going to race in the Millions Mile Saturday night. That was the top race on the grounds with a purse of $3 million. She was going to race against the top horses in the world. Oh, I forgot to mention that she was the only filly in the race. Dad felt she was the sharpest horse we had, and that's where she belonged. Fillies can beat colts but it was rare.

Stephanie and Dad watched as I worked my way down Rio's leg. I carefully palpated every tendon and manipulated every joint. Mom had reached Dr. Follansby on her cell phone. She was our main vet and would be here in about an hour or so. I knew how to examine most horses but past the exam part I was worthless. I would not want an equine vet taking care of the kids at the school. I sure as hell was not going to provide vet care to a million-dollar horse.

My exam revealed nothing. We walked her again. Dead lame. Dad, Stephanie and I went to work getting the other horses jogged. Mom stayed with Rio. No one spoke. We were sick. You have to own horses to understand. Sure, we might not be able to race this week and that might lose us the school. But that was not as important as Rio being well. The horse always came first.

I thought Dr. Follansby would block her. Starting with her foot and working her way up to her knee, injecting lidocaine in various places. I thought she would walk her around after each injection until she didn't limp anymore. The first injection that worked would tell us the source of the lameness.

Well, I scored no points for that guess. She came in and we all hovered around. She gave us the Azzie eyes. That meant she wanted some space. Mom assisted her while the other three of us pretended to work while we snuck peaks into the stall.

She did the same things I did but I knew she did them better. She asked Mom to twitch Rio's nose. She carefully put the wire loop around her upper lip and twisted it. Rio didn't mind too much. Dr. Follansby had to do a few things that Rio might not like, she wanted her and everyone to be safe. The twitch would take care of that.

A few more pokes and prods and then she left the stall and went to her truck. She returned with metal tongs that looked a little like bolt cutters. I recognized them as "hoof testers." She pulled a horseshoe off and applied the testers in various locations. The tester applied great pressure to a small spot. On the third area she tested Rio freaked. If it wasn't for the nose twitch, who knows what would have happened.

Dr. Follansby never flinched. She just chuckled. "Had you all going, didn't she? Just popping a gravel."

Goofiest ass thing I ever saw. Popping a gravel to a horse is kind of akin to having an infected hangnail. Hurts like hell if you touch it but, in the end, it is usually nothing. Of all the things that can make a horse dead lame popping a gravel had the best prognosis.

Dad had to know. "Will she be able to train and race?"

Follansby thought for a moment before answering. "Nothing until we get the abscess to pop. We will try the old-school methods today. You know, drawing salve, etc. Mrs. Zander, you know the drill. If she doesn't drain by tomorrow, I will ultrasound her and try to needle the abscess. I would prefer her to do it on her own, but we may need to get aggressive. Once the gravel pops, we can decide about training and racing."

Dad shifted to another subject. "Will she be in heat this Saturday?"

Dr. Follansby nodded. "I gave her the hormones on schedule to induce her. Why in the hell would you breed her on race day?"

Dad chuckled. "Who said anything about breeding her?"

CHAPTER 63

Always Hope School

Krenshaw, NJ

0900 August 19

Father Jonathan didn't think he could get up the tree but he did. It was the perfect spot to observe the parking lot for the school. The bishop was going to be super mad but what could he do? After getting ready to meet the bishop he got a very sick feeling in his stomach. Jenny was to meet the nurse at the school. On the surface it didn't seem like much, but something really bothered him about it. He called the bishop's secretary and told her he had Covid. He wondered just how long he had extended his time in purgatory with a lie to the bishop. Nothing to do now except follow through.

Shortly before his tree-climbing adventure, he had found a great picture of Myra Destefano RN at an awards ceremony for employees of Supreme Medical. She was being presented an award by Deuce. In and of itself, that was no big deal. He was the CEO, and they do stuff like that. But something bugged him about the picture. He did his best to follow up on his hunch then he decided to text me.

"Call me if you can."

Ten seconds later, his phone buzzed. Thankfully, he had silenced it prior to climbing the tree.

"ZZ," he whispered.

"Yes, Father," I whispered back. "Are you in the confessional?"

"Cut the shit ZZ. I got a bad feeling and I need your help."

"Sorry, go ahead."

Father Jonathan went on to inquire about everything I knew about Myra Destefano. He knew that I had hired her.

I relayed to him how lucky I was to find her. A short time ago she had responded to an employment website that I had posted a position on. I had a vacancy to fill, and I had a few nibbles. But no one had the creds I wanted until Myra appeared.

She had been a schoolteacher. Special needs kids of all things. From there, she got her BSN in nursing and had worked in the Pediatrics Department of Supreme Medical. She interviewed marvelously. She said she wanted to combine all her skills and thought that the Always Hope school was the way to do that. She was hoping to pursue a doctorate in nursing and was hoping to use the school to help with her thesis.

"What did you have to pay her?" Father inquired.

"That's the best freaking part. She came dirt cheap. She said that money was not as important to her as achieving her dreams and long-term goals."

"Did she feed Mr. G?"

"NOOOOOOOOO, what the hell is the matter with you? Shouldn't you be pissing off the bishop and not me? I would never have sex with an employee."

Father spoke very softly. "I am sending you a link to a picture. Tell me what you think."

I stared at the picture but saw only a CEO presenting an award to a nurse. Sure, it was Deuce and Myra but so what?

"Nothing special in that picture to me."

"ZZ, isn't it amazing that at this critical time in the history of your family, farm and school that someone with her talents just happens to find out about your position? And that someone agrees to a salary that is about 30% of what she probably had been making? Are you that lucky?"

"OK, I hit a homer. What about it?"

"Well, I thought I saw some bedroom eyes in that picture. You know how you look at the women you have been fornicating with."

"Father, you embarrass me."

"You know what I mean. Ms. Myra and Deuce had those eyes in that picture. At least I thought so. So, on a lark I sent PC the link. He confirmed that Deuce and Myra are an item. He has seen them in the owner's club at the track on multiple occasions. The last time was just a week ago. Plenty of PDA, etc."

"Shit, shit, she is to meet with Jenny today!!!"

"I know buddy. My big ass is close to breaking a branch on a tree outside the school. Get a hold of Joe and get over here. Don't come in but position your truck out of sight past the front entrance."

An hour later a large blue Ford truck pulled into the parking lot of the school. It parked behind the roll-off garbage dumpster. That was just fifteen feet from the base of the tree containing Father Jonathan. The window tint at first obscured the identity of the driver. But when he opened the window to toss his cigarette butt, Father recognized Knuckles. He texted me.

"Knuckles arrived in blue truck. He is parked behind the dumpster outside of camera site. Something is going down. Be ready."

The back door of the school opened. Jenny walked out in front of Myra. Father did not see a gun but the way they were walking was exactly the way someone would be brought out at gunpoint. They got to the dumpster and Knuckles jumped out of his truck. He grabbed Jenny. Then he covered her mouth and shoved her to the ground. Myra gagged her as Knuckles zip-tied her. They lifted her into the back seat of the crew cab.

Father texted Joe and me, "Jenny taken prisoner, bound and gagged in back of blue truck."

I was up for this. I had about enough of these cocksuckers. "Ready for a good time."

Knuckles drove slowly out the gate and turned right. He began to accelerate when he saw a flash of light on the right side of the road. That was followed by a loud crash. His truck spun out of control. He hit head-on into a tree at a very low speed. He wasn't hurt.

Before he could assess the cause of the incident or the extent of damage, the driver's side window exploded. As he worked feverishly to clear shards of glass from his face, he heard a shot from the back seat. The windshield exploded. Then the passenger window blew out and both doors opened. Before Knuckles could get his weapon out Joe had him out of the truck and on the ground. Knuckles never knew what hit him. He was out cold.

Jenny had head-butted Myra, who inadvertently discharged her weapon at the front windshield. Myra was dazed when I pulled her from the truck. Joe administered a pistol whip to the back of her head. She joined Knuckles deep in LA LA Land.

"Jenny, are you OK?" Father Jonathan asked as he removed the gags and ties.

"I am now but I was scared. I think they intended to kill me."

Joe interrupted. "No time for social soliloquy. We have to get our asses out of here before we have to answer a lot of questions for the cops. Jenny, take Knuckle's truck to the end of the road and find a place to keep it out of view. Wipe off any prints. When you are finished go back to the farm."

Jenny agreed. "Done."

We finished binding and gagging Myra and loaded both unconscious victims into the back of my truck.

I turned to Joe as he seemed to be running the show. "What are we going to do now?"

Joe grinned. "We are going to question these pieces of shit."

"I wonder where?" I said laughing.

Father Jonathan joined in. "I never thought I would be happy to see that place again. I guess it's just like the realtors say, location, location, location. This time I will be looking down!"

CHAPTER 64

Krenshaw Municipal Sewage Plant
1400 August 19

I started the party. "Time to wake them up."

Father Jonathan gleefully dumped a large bucket of brown water and fecal material onto the victims.

Joe encouraged their attention. "Hey shitheads, and I mean that literally, wake up."

Myra woke first and started to cry before she vomited profusely. She began to scream, and that woke Knuckles from his slumber.

Joe shouted at her. "Myra, listen to me. Padre here will drown you in water and shit if you don't shut up."

She stopped screaming.

"Good, now Knuckles, we are going to ask you some questions."

"Fuck you, asshole!" came Knuckle's response.

"Father please elicit Mr. Knuckles' cooperation."

Father dumped another bucket of the rancid mixture. A large turd came to rest on the top of Knuckle's head. He shook his head but it stuck there.

"What do you want?" Knuckles had decided to cooperate, at least temporarily.

I knew we were under some time constraints. "They are due for shift change here shortly, so we don't have much time. What did you have to do with my dad's accident."

Knuckles retorted, "Nothing, the asshole was drunk, and you guys got him off with your ties to the governor."

Another bucket of gaga went flying. Myra got one too, just for emphasis.

Myra gasped through vomiting episodes. "I didn't do anything, please stop with the crap."

She wanted to talk so I gave her a chance. "Why did you kidnap Jenny?"

No response. Both got another feculent shower.

I whispered to Joe. "Maybe they don't know anything, we better get a move on."

I turned my attention back to the detainees. "What's the number to the office?"

Myra was not on the same page. "What office?"

"Not you, slut. Knuckles, what's the number to the secret office that everyone knows about?"

Joe added. "Before you swear at us, be ready for another dousing."

Myra cried but Knuckles gave in. "201-477-9232."

Joe was pleased. "Very good. Last question. Did you kill Vucovich?"

No answer. We hadn't expected one. Father Jonathan gave them a final blessing then Joe flipped the switch that started the rotors. We fist-bumped as we walked to the truck. We jumped in and sped off. I dialed the number.

"Hello, this is Confidential Solutions."

"Yes, this is Dustin Stinker from the sewage treatment plant."

"Who…what?"

"Hey Deuce, we have two large pieces of crap down here at the sewage treatment plant that belong to you. We have to charge you extra this month."

"Zander you little asshole, what do you want?"

"A deal Deuce, a deal."

"What kind of deal?"

I laid it out for him. We had the picture of Jenny. I told him how we thought it had been made and he had no comment. I then went on to tell him that, in our opinion, the picture was equally damaging to Jenny as it was to Knuckles.

"What do you propose?"

"We destroy the picture, and you leave Jenny alone."

"What else did you take from this office?"

"Nothing, just the picture. But before I forget, thanks for the $100,000 for papering your horse. That will add to our pool of money for the entry fees."

"Don't mention it. How will I know the picture is destroyed?"

"You won't. Any more than we will know that you won't come after Jenny again."

"Sounds like a stalemate."

"Do we have a deal?" I knew I had him.

"Yes. Enjoy a win today because by the end of the week, I will own your farm and your precious Always Hope. You and your family will be shit out of luck. That pack of retards in that school of yours will be going back to the slums they came from."

I was livid. "Talk is cheap. See you at the track."

Joe made a fist and a vow. "I will make him eat those words about the kids, so help me God."

Father Jonathan concurred. "I'll ask him."

I told Deuce where to find Myra and Knuckles. We drove back to the farm.

On the way home, I asked Joe and Father. "They know we have the picture. Do you think they know about the CIC accounts or the Favors book?"

Joe didn't think so. "Azzie was 99% sure she sanitized the area. I had coached her what to look for. Luckily, she noted two hairs on the side of the book, one hair stuck to the computer keyboard, and one on the computer on-switch before she accessed them. She took close-up pictures and placed the hairs back in place when she was done. My guess is that they think we only knew about the picture, and that is all we got."

I couldn't believe it. "Do people really rely on shit like that?"

Joe grinned. "Yeah, particularly when they think they are invulnerable."

CHAPTER 65

Deuce sent a security officer to reclaim Myra and Knuckles. The officer made them ride in the back of the large SUV that he had fortunately covered with plastic before picking them up. On Deuce's orders, when they arrived back at the hospital, he parked outside the emergency department. Myra and Knuckles were required to go through the decontamination shower that was used for hazmat emergencies. Deuce met Knuckles in the men's changing room. He had fresh scrubs and a cup of coffee waiting.

"Was it necessary for us to use the decontamination showers? That water is pretty damn cold." Knuckles asked as he toweled off while pointing to his shriveled manhood.

"You are lucky that I didn't leave you there."

"What did you do with Myra?"

"I put her to bed without her supper. Bad girl. I probably should have spanked her too." Deuce laughed. "I sent her home. We have work to do. What did you find out?"

Knuckles sipped the coffee. "As we suspected during the 'power outage' last Saturday, no doubt caused by Zander et al, someone accessed the office. I found that the cold air return vent had been taped into position with fake screws. I suspect they had entered via the morgue."

Deuce continued the questioning. "Wasn't that the night they found the sick-assed coroner dead?"

"Same one. I can't relate the two."

"Nothing on the security tapes?" Deuce inquired.

"Of course, the cameras not on the life safety branch were useless. The hall cameras showed nothing. If they accessed the office via the vent, they wouldn't show anything."

"That's all you have?" Deuce erupted.

Knuckles objected. "Hey, don't use that tone with me. We go back too far, and we each know way too much about the other."

Deuce recanted. "Sorry, things were going so well. Then old man Zander got out. ZZ won his appeal. Jenny struck out and most likely has switched sides. We lost $100,000 last Saturday, and the office has been compromised. I think I am entitled to be upset."

Knuckles was somewhat sympathetic. "But not at me. There is some good news."

Deuce needed some. "ALL EARS"

Knuckles continued. "It appears that the computer was not accessed."

Deuce was skeptical. "How do you know that?"

"I employed a very low-tech sleuth trick to detect if the computer was disturbed. I placed two hairs in very inconspicuous places on the on-switch to the computer, and the port. They weren't disturbed. No one touched those things or anything else in the office. I am confident of that."

Deuce smiled. "So, they got the picture and missed the really good stuff?"

"Looks that way."

"Maybe this week will turn out well after all. I got two new contracts today. A hockey player and an Olympic swimmer. Not mega deals, mind you, but three or four times what we lost to Zander. We will get that back a thousand times over. Buy you a drink?"

CHAPTER 66

Fired Up Farms
1800 August 19

Stephanie said hello to the group and bolted for the track. She planned on spending the night rubbing Rio's foot and applying heat. She was beside herself. Keeping her busy was better than her chanting in some corner. Jenny also was on her way out the door when I stopped her.

"Jenny, you have proven yourself. You don't have to leave. As far as I am concerned you are one of the group. You can stay." All heads bobbled up and down in silent agreement.

Jenny blushed. Her voice cracked as she started to speak. "Thank you all. It means a lot to me that you would allow me to stay. But I think I can best serve everyone if I get over to the school. I suspect that Myra spent more time trying to gather information on the farm and the horses than she did taking care of kids. With your permission ZZ, I would like to access the files and see what's been happening for the past couple months."

I was impressed. "Wow, I never thought about that. Would you? Thanks."

After Jenny left, Mom and Dad explained about the lameness. There were some hurdles we might face getting Rio to race. But they ended their story with smiles on their faces. In the end they knew she would be ok. And to them, that was the most important thing.

Father Jonathan, Joe and I recalled our fun-filled afternoon. Azzie was pleased to hear that we had taken Myra and Knuckles to the sewage treatment plant. She was positively giddy. I summed things up by telling the group that Deuce and I came to an agreement about the picture. I personally felt we should destroy it. There was nothing there to prove Knuckle's connection. The picture of Jenny did show that Vucovich was dead before she was injured. Since we knew the murder scene had been staged, but could not prove it, the group agreed. Azzie took point on speaking with Dan as to best way to handle the picture so that no one was accused of tampering with evidence. That left the final order of business.

I had to know but I wasn't sure if I wanted to. "OK, Azzie, how do we stand financially?"

Azzie ran down the numbers. "We did not meet our goals coming into this week. We did ok, but I would have liked to have had more cash firepower."

Cash on hand is $2,100,000.

Debt to Crinelli construction and Azzie Huggins $900,000.

Joe looked sheepish. "Sorry guys. I've got audits coming up. I need to have that money back before then. With my family's previous connections, the feds are always trying to prove that we are laundering money or hiding income. The shit will really hit the fan if I am 500k short."

Azzie was apologetic. "Likewise, everyone. I stretched …."

I cut her off in mid-sentence. "Azzie, Joe, you have done as much as you can. I for one cannot let you ruin your lives and careers. I vote we put the $900,000 aside and try to work the $1,200,000 into what we need.

Azzie and Joe started to protest when Dad stood. "ZZ speaks for the Zander family, case closed. We thank you but we will find another way."

Azzie relented. "OK, but you know we need $7 million?"

Dad remained standing. "You all have a copy of our entries for Saturday. We have a number of horses and drives for ZZ Wednesday through Friday. If we can win, or finish second, in half of those we should generate around $600,000. That means we need to net around $4.5 million Saturday. Keep in mind that we can either win or finish second to a Supreme horse and we will get the winner's share when the drug positives are revealed.

Please refer to the chart on your handout. I laid out how much we were required to bet and how much we could potentially net on each race."

I was the first to speak. "I want to be sure my math is right. Am I correct that we will need to net around $4 mil on Rio's race?"

Dad concurred. "That's correct."

PC sounded skeptical. "If we get $1.5 mil for the purse, we need to make $2.5 mil betting? From what I remember the Supremes won $1.5 million betting last year, and that was a track record."

Dad smiled. "You remember correctly."

Joe was sullen. "How do we exceed that by a mil? ZZ's a great driver and Rio is a great horse. The two of them together won't generate much in way of odds. We could fire in everything we got and still come up short."

Dad shocked everyone. "That's why ZZ's not driving her."

I was incredulous. "Whoaaaaaa, you can't be serious!"

CHAPTER 67

Barn 7

Miracle Mile Racetrack and Casino

0900 August 20

Tim Dempster was right on time. He hopped on a 5 AM flight to Philly. He drove an hour and half to the track arriving at 9 AM as he promised. He met Dad outside the track cafeteria. Dad had arranged to borrow one of the blacksmith shops for a half hour.

Tim smiled. "Hey bud."

Tim called everyone bud. He had a smile on his face. He wasn't a large man. Just average size but if you look up sinewy in the dictionary you will find his picture. Not an ounce of fat on him. Forearms and biceps made of steel. The skin on his hands was tougher than steel. He dropped a cigarette butt to the ground, smashed it with his boot, and thrust his hand out to Dad.

Dad cringed a little from the firm grasp. "Tim, thank you so much for coming. How are your brothers and mom?"

Tim responded. "All well in Bridgeville, are you ready?"

As they walked to the blacksmith shop Dad explained the situation to Tim. "This filly popped a gravel at 4 AM. I need to train her today for her race Saturday, and I need you to work your magic."

"OK, bud, let's take a look."

Tim did a thorough exam of all four feet. He used his own hoof testers on all the hoofs and let out a satisfied grunt. He then went to work on the affected foot, creating a pad to protect the frog (sole) of the foot and then he applied a thin shoe. He applied matching thin shoes to the other three feet and lit up a cigarette.

"You can train her in these today, but I want you to pull them after she is done. Stall rest her Thursday and Friday. I will be back Saturday morning to do her up for the race."

"You don't have to."

Tim wouldn't hear it. "Hey bud, I wouldn't miss it for the world."

Tim took off for the airport and Stephanie walked Rio back to her stall. Stephanie was pumped.

"Uncle Timmy fixed you up big girl. Now let's get to work."

Wednesday night was fun. It was two finger night. My first thought was to jog in front of the Supremes and flip them double birds. That wasn't what two finger night was about, but it made me laugh. The reality was that this was a $100,000 race and anyone was free to enter. The only caveat was that the drivers could only use two fingers to drive. That was an expression trainers and drivers used to describe a dream horse that was easy to control. "You can drive her with two fingers." That meant you didn't need your whole hand around each line, just one index finger on each hand.

For tonight's race every driver had to wear special gloves that only allowed them to drive with the two permitted fingers. The chance of a driver losing control of his horse was high, but the purse was high too for the caliber of horse entered.

Dad had entered Fired Up Jackie, and she was a perfect fit for the race. As the gate pulled, we left for the front with purpose and never looked back. There was a minor wreck at the half mile pole. Apparently one of the horses needed more control than what the driver could provide with two fingers. But as the saying goes, "that was behind us." We pocketed $50,000. After a few other wins we tallied $200,000 for the evening. We were on track.

CHAPTER 68

Fired Up Farms
0400 August 23

No one could sleep. We were all up by 4 AM. Thank God there was daylight racing on Millions Day. I don't think any of us could take waiting for a 7 PM first post. I was happy with how we were positioned going into the day. Thursday turned out as expected. We lost the big race to the Supremes. Their horse was a monster. With the "go juice" that we were sure he got, he was unbelievable.

We won a few others races and I won the chariot race. I would have been crucified in that race except for the training I got during the week. Just like in Rome, it was MMA and harness racing all rolled together in one. Blue Balls took a swing at me with his whip. I had been alerted to be ready for that tactic. Just like I practiced, I grabbed it in midair and pulled as hard as I could. I nearly yanked him out of his bike. I decorated his surprised face with a large collection of my oral secretions and left him in the dust.

My trainer was none other than Billie "Cha-Ching" Browner. Yes, Billie. He showed up at the farm two weeks ago. He had been screwed over by Deuce and wanted to help us. And help us he did. Billie knew a ton of stuff about Millions Week. Things had changed a lot in the three years that I had been absent from driving. The chariot lessons he gave me were incredibly helpful. But we spent the most time practicing what Billie called "A-A-A Gap." Now, there was something interesting about how Billie pronounced it this week. Billie only stuttered out three As when saying "A Gap." Normally, he was good for 5-10 As.

Last week Billie and I had stopped to see some members of the Army with the horses we were working. Jenny was there with the kids and their therapists. I introduced Billie to Jenny, and he stuttered himself into a tizzy. Jenny patiently let him finish and asked one of the therapists for her opinion.

Boom, boom, boom, the therapist tells Billie she might be able to help him. And damn if she didn't improve him some in just a week. The less he stuttered, the prouder he was of himself. I never realized, until he told me while we were jogging horses, how bad the stuttering made him feel about himself. I would never have believed that cocky little bastard had low self-esteem. For a doctor I'm dimwitted sometimes. God help the other harness drivers in the country when Billy musters more self-confidence.

Friday brought the ostrich races. I fell off mine. Maybe Billie and I should have spent a little more time on that. I might as well have fallen off my drives too as I had a horrible night. I had two minor wins, but the big Mo, (momentum), was gone. I got an earful from the fans at the rail. "Asshole", "Fuck you ZZ", "Eat shit." I went to the driver's room and watched the replays. All I could think was "Asshole," "Fuck you ZZ," and "Eat shit."

This morning no one else was permitted in the kitchen. Jenny and Azzie made that absolutely clear. You don't mess with them. Powerful women, a force to be reckoned with. So, the rest of us waited impatiently.

At the appointed time the door to the dining room opened and nothing short of a spectacle appeared. A long, well-appointed table was beautifully adorned with fresh cut flowers. Place settings of priceless china and Waterford crystal completed the ambiance.

"Mimosa's anyone?" Azzie inquired. "ZZ excluded, of course."

Mom, Dad, Stephanie, Joe, Father Jonathan, Jenny, Billie, PC, Dan and Tim Demptser picked their beverages and took their assigned seats.

Even though Jenny had been cooking she looked absolutely stunning in a white dress and high heels. I caught Billie eye humping her.

Jenny smiled at him as she raised her mimosa and addressed the group. "My friends, here we are at the precipice. We win or we lose. Now we all know that we can only win if we save our souls. But maybe we can do both. Today we take on Satan, Supreme Stables. If we are going to win, we must start out strong. Welcome to a victor's breakfast. Father, please lead us in prayer."

Father Jonathan was ready. "Dear Lord, look at your flock that we serve. The little ones who have physical or mental handicaps that make them vulnerable to our society. Help us to help them."

"Amen." I shouted. I was ready to eat.

Azzie and Father Jonathan gave me the eyes.

Father Jonathan continued. "Dear God, you created us, and you created Fired Up Frat Boy, Supreme Taco, Wicked Fast, Fired Up Alabama and Fired Up Rio. Let your grace shine upon them and ZZ today as we head into battle. We thank you for the opportunity to make a difference in the lives of the children. We thank you for the great gifts of friends and friendships that you have bestowed upon us. We especially thank you for allowing us to love our previous enemies, Jenny and Billie, and welcome them now as friends. Amen."

And then we got to eat. Great meal it was. Fitting of a grand buffet at Caesar's Palace in Las Vegas. Tons of fresh fruit, bagels and lox, omelets made to order, sausage patties, fried potatoes, assorted pastries, and tons of coffee.

Tim wanted to get to the track. He was anxious to see how Rio's foot looked. So were we. He took off with Stephanie. Mom and Dad followed. I thought I had to stay for the bettor's meeting called by PC, but he dismissed me. "ZZ you just win every race and we will take care of the rest." That was a tall order. I saw in the program that I was still programmed to drive Rio. What the heck was Dad up to?

PC started the meeting with Joe, Azzie, and Father Jonathan by going over betting procedures first. Normally betting pools were closed when the gate opened and the race began. Millions Week was a whole other animal. Not only were the owners required to bet a minimum on their horse, betting continued until the horses reach the $5/8$ poles. And the drivers were wired for sound. The owners, and any fans who wanted to buy the frequency required, were able to hear the drivers.

Joe was incredulous. "You gotta be shitting me. That's crazy. Being allowed to bet after the race is half over."

Father Jonathan responded. "You can bet all kind of sporting events after they start. I've bet football games into the fourth quarter. The odds reflect the score at the time."

Joe laughed. "Betting from your own pocket or out of the collection plate?"

That earned Joe a Zander salute. The group laughed. It was good to help ease the anxiety they were experiencing.

PC explained further. "Well, it's different, and a lot of times the horse on the lead just runs away with it. So, the leader in the race usually gets most of the action. That of course drives the odds way down. But if you like a horse that comes from behind you can get some decent odds. It's hard for most people to bet a horse that is last at the ½ mile pole, especially in good races."

Joe thought he had an angle. "But the drivers know. We just listen to them and bet accordingly? Right?"

PC continued the educational session. "Some drivers are better than others at being realistic. I mean if their horse is dead, you won't hear a word out of them. But it's not uncommon for three or four drivers to be screaming at their owners to bet as they hit the half mile pole."

He recommended that they bet 50% of their money on Frat Boy in the third race, and that they do it before the start. I was supposed to leave with him and park anyone that pulled. Dad wanted Frat Boy, "on the engine," as harness race lingo goes. That meant he was to lead the race the whole way. PC expected the Supremes to bet Supreme Court heavily, which would raise the odds on Frat Boy.

He was worried that Taco and Wicked Fast might not be good enough to win. He said that he would take care of what was to be wagered on them. If we won with Frat Boy, he felt everyone should bet 25% of what they had on Alabama. He recommended betting half of what they had for the race before the start. The other half should be laid in if she was better than fourth at the quarter pole.

"If everyone is cool with things so far, we can turn to the twelfth race."

Joe had a question. "How does Rio's foot play into the equation? I mean she was dead lame. How can she win a race?"

PC smiled. "Actually, that helps us significantly. Although there is no guarantee that she can race, the odds are that she can. Popping a gravel can be overcome quickly. But the knowledge of that happening can make people nervous about betting her."

"But only we know," Azzie added.

PC corrected her. "Unfortunately, the whole backside knows. There are eyes and ears everywhere. We must assume that everyone other than John Q Public knows about her foot. But what they don't know is that Tim Dempster is a master, and Carl Zander is no slouch. If they put her on the track, she is ready to race. That is our edge."

He went on to request that under no circumstances was anyone to bet on Rio before the race started. He recommended that they have their full bet loaded onto the phone, tablet or whatever betting device they were using. They were to hit send after she passed the half mile pole if she was first or second. Then he emphasized that meant first or second REGARDLESS of whether she was at the pylons or parked out.

Father spoke up. "Carl mentioned something about ZZ not driving her. Will Billy be in the bike?"

PC shook his head. "Carl would not tell me. But Billie can't drive until Millions Week is over. He signed a bad contract with Deuce. But Carl, being closed-mouthed, tells me that he has something wild planned that he doesn't want anyone to get wind of before the race. It should be exciting."

CHAPTER 69

Miracle Mile Racetrack and Casino
1230 August 23

"Ladies and gentlemen, the management, staff, and horseman of Miracle Mile Racetrack and Casino welcome you to this year's edition of Millions Saturday. The greatest spectacle in all of harness racing. Please stand for the national anthem. If you can stand, and don't want to stand, get the hell out." Gabe Vatter, the track announcer, was as wired up as every trainer, driver, owner and fan.

"Please welcome Milly Anderson, a groom for the Supreme Stables, to sing the anthem."

Milly stood tall and proud, and delivered a powerful rendition of the anthem. At the conclusion of the last note there was a flyover of F-18 jets, followed a minute later by a flyover in the opposite direction. Whatever anyone did in the past was doubled or tripled on Millions Saturday.

Gabe keyed his mike. "Now ladies and gentlemen please remain standing as we honor horseman who this year crossed the finish line of life."

Bagpipes played as a parade of identical black Mercedes drove down the stretch. On the roof was a placard with the name of the deceased. Inside the vehicles were their relatives and friends. As each car slowly passed the tote board a picture of the honoree was displayed on the 100 x 50 foot video screen along with a lifetime achievement summary. There were trainers, drivers, owners and even some track employees honored. The final car stopped at the winner's circle.

Gabe informed the crowd. "Ladies and gentlemen, our final salute goes to Ken Harrow, who was tragically killed in an auto accident this year. Celeste Harrow, his widow, is accompanied by her son Carl Adam Harrow and family friend Carl Zander.

Celeste handed the baby to Carl. She in turn was handed an urn that had been sitting on a table in the winner's circle.

A microphone was held in her direction as she opened the urn and spread the ashes in the winner's circle. "Ken you will always be a winner to me, and both Carls. Rest in peace my love. Now let's see some racing!"

Tim Dempster was satisfied with Rio's foot. Pretty damn close to fully healed. For today close would have to do. The other job he had to do later scared him a little. He didn't know Azzie well, but he did come to learn that it was damn difficult to say no to her. Dad just raised his eyebrows when he heard. Mom thought it was just awesome. Tim preferred to get it done at the last minute in the paddock.

Dad inquired of Tim. "Did you pad that foot well?"

Tim could barely stifle a laugh. "Yeah bud, really good."

On the way to the track, they had decided that if Rio's foot was good, they would give the nosey people at the track some misinformation. By padding her foot a little aggressively, it was hoped that she would look a little gimpy jogging in her warmup. A problem that would be totally corrected when Timmy removed the padding and reset her shoes before the race.

I was in the driver's room when the announcer gave out the list of scratches and driver changes. As usual, there were very few of each. Everyone wanted their horse to race and every driver worth his salt wanted their chance to drive. I was shocked not to hear about a driver's change for the 12th race on Rio. Dad couldn't have been clearer that I wasn't driving her. I thumbed through the program for the hundredth time. I had not noticed the back cover until now. It was a full-page picture of Azzie and some of our kids smearing lipstick on her. "Good Luck to Fired Up Farms." Azzie Huggins and the employees of Exquisite Evolutions.

I warmed up Frat Boy, then Taco, and then Wicked Fast. All seemed to be in good shape and not too keyed up except for Wicked

Fast. He tried to run off two or three times. Luckily, he calmed down each time he passed the Army. The whole gang had camped out in their usual location at the top of the stretch.

It was hard to see as I was going by, but there was a small man walking beside Father Jonathan. Most people looked small beside him. Both had a large cardboard container filled with pink and blue cotton candy. You know, like the vendors use at the ball game. I could have sworn that was the bishop with Father Jonathan. Good thinking Padre, he can't chew your ass too much in front of the kids.

I had nothing in the first race but I watched it intently on the monitor. There was some serious racing going on. Bumping, jostling, changing course abruptly, the whole nine yards. Today there were no steward inquiries. Let em' play was the moto.

Frat Boy was still keyed up in the post parade. I told PC that he was keyed up. He told me to take an enema and just drive. I watched the tote board blink and change. Man, the money was rolling in on us. I was half hoping our people weren't betting most of it. This horse had me a little worried. My thoughts were interrupted by the Blue Man on Supreme Dream.

"ZZ that flea bag looks keyed up. Maybe you should give him a Xanax or something."

"Fuck you and the horse you rode in on," I screamed as we turned our horses. Then I said calmly into the mike. "PC, fire it in, fire it in!"

We had the five hole and Blue Man had the two. I saw him looking down the line to see who was leaving. I purposely had Frat Boy two lengths off the gate. I could hear PC ,"ZZ, WTF?"

I let Frat Boy take a good run at the gate even though that risked him hitting it before the start. Garry Vatter took over. "Fired Up Frat Boy nearly pushed the gate down leaving and grabs an easy lead. Up on the outside comes the Blue Man sending Supreme Dream forward. They are flying to the quarter. Just Plain Nasty is a distant third. The rest are just watching a good race."

Dad had wanted me to stay on the engine. But I knew if I parked Blue Man out that we would take all the action being bet from now until the ⅝ pole. Our betting income would take a big hit. I pulled back on the lines and let Blue Man go. Gary didn't let that pass. "Fired Up Stable blinks first as Supreme Dream rolls to the front. First quarter in a blistering 25.4."

I could hear Dad bitching in my ear, so I wanted to say something funny. All I could think of was "meanwhile back at the sand dune the Arabs were busy eating their dates."

PC said "what????"

Stephanie was laughing, and so was I.

Knowing the Blue Man like I did, and given Billie's sage advice, I knew that Blue Man would roll to around the ⅜ pole. So, there was no sense pulling now. I had to wait to just before the half. His tendency was to try to rest his horse from the 3/8ths to the ⅝ or ¾ pole, and then roll him on home. Well, I planned to zig when he zagged.

"PC."

"Yes."

"Send it in, send it in!"

Our odds had climbed to 3 to 1. Azzie, Joe, PC and Father pounded away at their phones and betting devices. Just before the half I stoked up the Frat Boy and we flew down the backstretch. I had to clear before the ¾ pole or we were toast.

Gabe hit high C. "ZZ pops the plugs and gives Frat Boy his marching orders. Blue Man asks Supreme Dream for more steam. They are steppin' now!!!"

I shook the lines and ran my whip over Frat Boy's ass. He responded, showing his class. We cleared the Blue Man as I flipped him off.

"Fired Up Frat Boy clears. ZZ gives Blue Man that famous Zander Salute as he opens up on a tiring Supreme Dream. They round the turn and reach the top of the stretch. Fired Up Frat Boy is up by four lengths and digs for more. The Army encourages him on from the rail. It's all Fired Up Frat Boy to the wire. Mile in 150:2."

We had decided to have only two children and handlers for any winning picture, except for Rio's race. I turned Frat Boy around to go back for our picture and was overjoyed to see everyone else in the winner's circle. There were two children too, and they had special handlers. Father Jonathan approached me with his companion.

"ZZ, great race. I would like you to meet Bishop Carlucci."

"Bishop, it's my pleasure. Thank you for coming. It's a great honor for us, and I am sure the kids will never forget it.'

"God bless you son, keep going."

I have never met a bishop. I would have thought he was taller. What difference that would make I don't know. My head was full of all kinds of goofy thoughts.

PC interrupted my twisted thinking. "Net of $870k betting, good start, nice drive, but you had me worried."

"Show a little faith there's magic in the night, you ain't a beauty but hey, you're alright. And that's alright with me." I sang a horrible rendition of "The Boss," but I was having fun. Good things happen when I have fun. Most of the time.

CHAPTER 70

Miracle Mile Racetrack and Casino
1500 August 23

Taco's race went as expected. She gave it an impressive effort but Xanadu, a recent purchase by the Supremes ended her winning streak. I couldn't wait to see what all they found in her system. Luckily, PC had instructed everyone to cool it on betting the race. We only lost about $50,000 plus the $100,000 we were required to bet. Maybe that wasn't as lucky as I thought.

I was off until the seventh race, but I had horses to warm up. Alabama was her usual monster self. Big, beautiful, and an absolute beast. Stephanie had a smirk on her face when she pulled Rio out of the paddock stall. We walked out the door and I thought Rio looked a little gimpy.

I covered my mik as I quizzed Stephanie. "Is she ok?"

"Yeah, But I want to warm her up. I will warm her up easy. We are giving a show here."

It wasn't unusual for Stephanie to warm her up. The two of them were tight and Rio behaved better for her. I sipped my coffee and watched. Rio wasn't terrible, but she was pretty steppy gaited. I noticed it, and so would most horsemen. I was still a little worried, joke or no joke. When Stephanie got back, she told me that Rio would not be gong another warmup trip. She called the shots on the warmups.

"Am I still driving her?" I had to know.

"Far as I know," Stephanie replied as she got Rio ready for a nice bath.

Mom had Wicked Fast decked out to match my colors. I hooked my tricked-out racing bike to him. I would have used it earlier but Frat

Boy was too green to use it on, and Taco was too big. But it fit Wicked Fast. It had been specially made for me. There were all kinds of small LED lights powered by a tiny battery under the seat. It all had to be super lightweight, or it could cost me fifths of a second.

As we entered the track for the post parade, I started my light show. The white lights lit, and then went out, sequentially from the front of the back of the bike. The speed at which they went on and off were tied to my speed. The faster I went, the faster they went. I also had lights in the wheels, and on command they formed "Z" s in the spokes. And of course, the ZZ on my back blinked. None of this crap was legal during the regular season but today was different.

As we jogged down the stretch in the post parade, I saw the Army hanging on the rail. I lit the lights, and they went completely bonkers. They were pointing and laughing and screaming. I swear the bishop was screaming the loudest of all.

For this race I had the eight hole and Blue Man had the seven. I was planning on gunning out of there to find a position. I had no intention of cutting the mile but I had no intention of eating everyone's dust either. As we approached the gate the Blue Man suddenly drifted out toward me. Before I could react, I heard "whooossh." I knew right away what had whooshed. The prick had cut my tire.

No way could I win now.

"Abort, abort, abort!" I screamed into the mike in case anyone in our group had thought about betting. "Flat tire," I sighed.

We got away last, and I pulled up at the half. I showed the paddock judge the tire and he informed the judges in the judge's booth as to why I pulled up.

"Be more careful what you drive over ZZ," The judge said tongue in cheek.

He damn well knew that Blue Man had cut the tire. But Millions Week was Millions Week.

Tim Dempster removed the extra padding and put on the correct shoes. He then nervously drilled small holes in the front of Rio's four hoofs. He reached into his pocket and pulled out four, two-caret diamonds, and cemented them into the holes. At the same time Stephanie put diamond studs in Rio's pierced ears. Fired Up Rio looked like a couple million bucks. She was elegant by herself and the diamonds were worth a few million at least. Stephanie pulled her out of the stall so the USTA photographer could get pictures of "Diamond Rio." That was the title they gave her for this picture. The picture that would be featured on the cover of the October edition of their magazine, "Hoof Beats."

I won easily with Chantilly Lace and put a new lifetime mark on her.

Desmond Wallace was thrilled. "Great drive ZZ."

"I was just a passenger. She did all the work. She is a sweet filly. Do you want to sell her?"

"Jinxing me now!" he teased. "You know when you turn down an offer for a horse, how the horse always goes to shit."

That was a horsemen's wives' tale.

I reassured him. "That's why I never made you an offer. If you ever do want to sell her, I know Dad would be interested."

I found Dad waiting for me at Alabama's paddock stall.

"ZZ, are you ready?" he asked.

"I am, how is Alabama?"

Dad grinned. "A total monster, she is ready for however you chose to drive her."

"Good, because this race will be a little strange. And if Billy is right, she will need to be very drivable."

"Is there something I should know." Dad looked worried.

"You don't want to know anything, trust me."

The bugle sounded for the tenth race. We walked to the door of the paddock without speaking. Dad just nodded his head. That was his way of saying "I know you got this." I got the feeling I was going to drive Rio, but Dad hadn't said a word. That was strange.

No time to think about that now. Alabama was jumpy and I really needed her to calm down. I knew that she could leave, if needed, but it wasn't my best driving strategy.. When she left and got the lead she tended to lollygag around. She waited for horses to get close to her before she dug in. It was her way of messing with them. That was fine for races where she was hands over fist better than the rest. That wasn't the case tonight. She could beat these, but if she waited for them at the top of the stretch, they would go right on by.

Gabe introduced each horse as they paraded in front of the stands. We got some applause near the wire but that paled in comparison to the reception we got at the top of the stretch. I spied the bishop, with a kid in each arm, jumping up and down and screaming with them. Behind the bishop was Father Jonathan with two thumbs up in the air. It was all I could do to hold Alabama in check. When I did, I fired the light show for the kids. Another chorus of screams and chants erupted. I was as fired up as Alabama. It was time to kick some serious ass.

We settled in behind the gate. I was pleased to feel that Alabama was ready for me to drive her. I could tell. Sometimes she had no interest in doing what I wanted. But during the warmups she couldn't do enough to please me. So far, so good. I had her on the gait, but I had no intention of leaving. Good thing, because as the gate opened there was a calvary charge.

Vatter breathlessly described the situation. "It's a donnybrook. Five horses are leaving strong and battling for the lead. Hunka Hunka has her nose in front at the pylons. Mumblypeg looms large to her outside. Supreme Dream is third, but she is hung two-wide. Supreme Hilarious settles in fourth at the pylons. Big Nose is caught three-wide. Big Nose jumps it off, Big Nose is all boogered up on a serious break. They approach the quarter. Mumblypeg gets the top, but Supreme Dream powers up attempting to get to the front. Supreme Hilarious is now third. High Octane sits fourth. Fired Up Alabama is just fifth and showing no fire at all. Giggles is rough-gaited sixth, Hush Hush Hush is a quiet seventh. Big Nose is last. Supreme Dream grabs the front. ZZ lights a match under Fired Up Alabama and she responds. Mumblypeg stays at the rail behind Supreme Dream. Hilarious jumps in front of a charging Fired Up Alabama. ZZ grabs a big handful of leather to keep from running her over. In any other race that would be a foul, but all is fair during Millions Week. Supreme Dream opens a quick three length lead. Mumblypeg and Supreme Hilarious are racing side by side up the backstretch. ZZ can follow them and let Dream get away, or he can go three wide and lose tons of ground. What will he do? This race will be decided in the next ten seconds."

I opened Alabama's throttle as I approached the blocking horses. She never flinched, even though we were rapidly approaching a brick wall of horses. We had practiced hard for this moment, and now was the time to execute.

I opened my mike. "Fire, Fire, Fire!" I yelled as I popped the plugs out of Alabama's ears.

PC and the gang bet feverishly as I lined up my sights. It was just as Billy predicted. Dream was flying to the ¾ pole as the other two blocked. Not content with the inside blocking horse being at the pylons, they would likely be half a bike width off the pylons. I could go two and a half wide and lose a ton of ground, or I could follow Billie's advice. "You can aaaasssssfuckem by shooting the AAA Gap."

Vatter painted the picture. "Supreme Dream keeps to her business on the front. Mumblypeg and Supreme Hilarious set up a blocking scheme the Eagles would be proud of. ZZ sends Fired Up Alabama dead at them. He has only two choices, go three wide, or sit tight. There is going to be a collision!!!"

I remember thinking, "OK Billie, I hope this works." The A gap was in between the pylons and Mumblypeg. As predicted the gap was not big enough for my bike to fit through. If I got inside the pylons I would likely be disqualified. I closed my eyes and violently shifted my weight to the right as Billie had shown me. With the left tire in the air we aimed at the A gap.

Vatter went wild. "Holy shit, holy shit, ZZ got his bike onto one wheel. He snuck in between the pylons and Mumblypeg and is closing in on Supreme Dream. Unbelievable."

I let Alabama settle in behind Supreme Dream. She knew what to do. She chomped on Blue Man's helmet. Right about now he realized he was screwed. I pulled her as we passed the Army. The lights were blinking so fast that they looked solid white. I executed a perfect double Zander salute, and she exploded.

Vatter was nearly out of breath. "Fired Up Alabama blasts down the lane, winning for fun. Amazing drive, amazing trotter, amazing Millions Week. It ain't over yet folks."

The winner's circle was absolute chaos. I counted at least ten kids and handlers. So much for limiting the visitors to two. The bishop was hoarse. Father Jonathan had broken his own face with a huge smile. Stephanie got beside me for the picture, and then she laid it on me.

"When you get back to the paddock Dad wants you to……."

"He what?"

"Just do it."

Back in the paddock Mom escorted Alabama to her stall until she could provide a urine sample for testing. I saw my opportunity in the hallway and took it.

"Ah shiiiiitttt!" I screamed as my boot slipped in a large pile of horse manure. I laid in the crap for a minute for effect.

People ran to help me up, but I refused.

"My back, my back, don't move me. Get the medics!" I screamed.

The medics arrived and strapped me to a backboard. Off we went to Supreme Medical. Knuckles got a call from the 911 dispatcher, who happened to be one of his asshole buddies.

"ZZ in ambulance heading to hospital with a back injury."

Knuckles started to tell Deuce when Vatter interrupted the conversation.

"Attention race fans, attention race fans. We have a late driver's change in the twelfth Race. Fired Up Rio will be driven by Stephanie Zander. ZZ was injured by a fall in the paddock. He is stable but has been taken to Supreme Medical for an evaluation. Provisional driver, Stephanie Zander will drive Fired Up Rio."

Deuce was pleased. "Isn't she one of those fucked up kids? Like the ones in their precious school."

Knuckles answered. "They say she has some kind of autism or some shit like that."

"Can she drive? I can't believe they didn't grab someone else. There are a ton of great drivers here without drives in the twelfth."

Knuckles was also puzzled. "That Carl Zander can be quite the asshole. But when we finish wiping them out after the Millions Mile, he won't have to worry about making good decisions. All he will have to decide is what time he wants to go the unemployment office each week."

"Look at the damn odds for Explosion, he's freaking $1/9$!"

Knuckles sighed. "That's not unexpected. The big-money guys aren't going to bet on a provisional driver. His odds may get a little better but we should look at exactas and trifectas to try to get some return."

In the back of the ambulance Amos chided me. "ZZ, you smell pretty bad, and you got my backboard all funky."

"Sorry Amos, I had to stage that fall and it seemed like a good idea at the time. You know what to do?"

"Yeah man, easier than last week. We drive to the hospital. When we get near there you refuse to go to that 'shitty hospital,' and you sign off. Jenny picks you up in the parking lot, and you get back to the track."

"I should be able to make it back in time to see the end of the race, but I won't be able to drive. It was Dad's idea and I have to respect it."

"Who's Dad? Do you mean Carl?" Amos had never heard me call Carl, "Dad".

"Carl is my dad, and I couldn't be a prouder son."

365

CHAPTER 71

Miracle Mile Racetrack and Casino
1800 August 23

The handle in the eleventh race was off by half compared to the projections. The oxygen was sucked out the room when my "accident" was announced. There was utter shock that SZ, (Stephanie), would now pilot Fired Up Rio in the biggest race in harness racing. The money poured in on Supreme Explosion. His odds initially plummeted but in the past few minutes he had risen to 1 to 2. He was still a very heavy favorite. One of the paddock reporters asked to interview Stephanie live. She declined, so they chased Dad down and tried to get some information from him. He agreed to the interview and answered the first question.

"First of all, I hope ZZ is alright. He took a pretty good spill. But no, I am not worried about Stephanie driving. Sure, she lacks experience, but I can't think of a better race to get some in." It was all Dad could do to keep a straight face.

The interviewer was incredulous. "You must be kidding me, this is the top purse race of the year. Even though she is your daughter, you have to admit that she is not qualified to drive in this race."

"Fuck you pal." Dad pushed the microphone away from his face and stormed off.

"Well Gary, sorry about the f bomb, but that's about all Carl had to say. Back to you." Dan Kindle signed off from the paddock.

Deuce looked at Knuckles. "Did Zander get to the hospital yet? I don't trust that asshole. It would be just like him to show up and drive at the last minute."

Knuckles held up one finger. "Hold one second. My dispatcher is on the line. Are you sure? Good."

Deuce was impatient. "C'mon, we don't have much time."

Knuckles reassured him. "Good news. He refused to go into 'that shitty hospital' and signed off. He is on his way back in a private vehicle."

Deuce wasn't so happy. "How is that good news?"

Knuckles explained. "He cannot drive tonight unless cleared at the nearest ER. He can't drive, case closed."

Deuce dialed his trainer, Hennesey. "How are things in the paddock?"

"Pretty good."

Deuce didn't like the answer. "What do mean, pretty good. WTF is that?"

"Your horse got a big boner."

"What, What? Are you drunk; you prick? If you are, I will strangle you with my bare hands."

"No boss, I think that Zander filly is in heat. All the boys in the race who still have their nuts are excited."

"Can't you put something up his nose?"

"We tried that. Remember the race where he was throwing his head all around and eventually, he broke stride?"

Deuce had to think a few seconds before he answered. "Yeah, what of it?"

"We put some stuff up his nose that day to block out the smell. It made him worse. Listen Tom, once we get out of the paddock he will settle down. I will have Blue Man keep him away from her in the post parade. With ZZ out I know we can easily get to the front. He won't smell anything behind him."

"He better not."

PC made an announcement to the betting crew. "Keep powder dry, nothing goes in till ⅜ pole."

I agreed. "Got it, boss."

"ZZ, is that you."

"Yep, I'm with the Army. Colors are off. I am ready to send it in."

Back in the paddock Dad had some last words with Stephanie.

Dad asked. "Any questions?"

"No Dad, thanks for believing in me."

Dad beamed. "Always did sweetie, I know you will do your best." The bugle sounded.

Vatter could hardly contain himself. "Ladies and gentlemen here is the field for our twelfth, and final race. The Miracle Millions ultimate event at a purse of three million dollars. Post position one belongs to Fired Up Rio. She's a three-year-old filly by Brazilian Bad Boy, out of the world champion mare, Always Hope. She is owned by The Fired Up Farms for the benefit of The Always Hope School. Carl Zander trains her. She has amassed earnings of $278,000 this year on only four starts. Tonight, she is adorned with six, two caret diamonds valued at four hundred thousand dollars each courtesy of Exquisite Evolutions. That's SZ not ZZ in the bike. Stephanie Zander making her first parimutuel drive."

I almost cried as they worked their way up the stretch toward The Army. The filly was dazzling, and then there was Stephanie. Beautiful smile on her face and she was as calm as could be. They were both amazing. Stephanie stopped her in front of the screaming Army. Rio knelt down on one knee and bowed her head. The diamonds in her ears flashed in the track lights. Stephanie pulled her to her feet. My ears hurt when the Army exploded in a mixture of screams and cries. Stephanie set the lights off and they slowly trotted into the turn.

Vatter introduced the rest of the horses, but I wasn't paying much attention. I had the binoculars up and focused on Supreme Explosion. He was a little lathered up. I carefully looked over the field. Hyphenated,

Quick Response and Playful Platypus didn't look all that promising on paper. Platypus was the longest odds. He had a bad post position and little gate speed. But I remembered seeing that horse swoop a field at Miami Valley Raceway in a stakes race. I found my second-place horse.

I know Dad wanted Stephanie to roll out of the gate. The problem was that it was damn difficult to roll out of the one-hole. That had to do with the slanted starting gate. The way it was slanted it kind of held the one-horse back. Rio had plenty of speed. If she had the five-hole, or so, I think she could outstep Supreme Explosion to the front. But starting from the far inside was dicey.

As they made their turns and moved in behind the starting gate it was clear that Explosion was still unsettled. Vatter ran down the field for the last time. Stephanie was singing as loudly as she could. It was "Rio", by Duran Duran.

Moving on the floor now, babe

You're a bird of paradise

Cherry ice cream smile

I suppose it's very nice

With a step to your left and a flick to the right

You catch that mirror way out west

You know you're something special

And you look like you're the best

Now Stephanie screamed:

Her name is Rio and she dances on the sand

Just like that river twisting through a dusty land

And when she shines, she really shows you all she can

Oh Rio, Rio dance across the Rio Grande

Stephanie finished the last words as the gate opened. Vatter took over.

"That's Fired Up Rio charging out and protecting her pylon position. Supreme Explosion leaves from the seven-hole with purpose. SZ asks Rio for more. As they reach the first turn Rio settles for second at the pylons. Supreme Explosion rumbles to the front. Hyphenated is third. Quick Response got away fourth. Lots of Speed didn't show much today and is fifth. Razmataz sixth, Supreme Cracker seventh, Our Baby eighth, and Playful Platypus can see them all.

They approach the quarter and damn if Stephanie Zander doesn't pull Fired Up Rio. Now that's a rookie miscue. She had the perfect two-hole trip behind the heavy favorite. SZ jiggles and joggles and Rio almost gets by. Supreme Explosion remains game at the pylons, but they are throwing down, big time. Quarter in 26 smoking seconds. Rio has a very tenuous lead but is going the long mile on the outside."

PC keyed his mike. "Fire, Fire, Fire!" Fingers clicked. Hundreds of thousands of dollars were wagered on Rio. I decided to put mine on the exacta with Rio first and Playful Platypus second. That rat was still sitting last when I heard Stephanie calmly talking to Rio.

"That's a girl, stay right there and give the big boy a good sniff of that cooze." Being somewhat dense I just figured out the plan. Dad had Rio brought into heat for the race. Stephanie had to position her to take Explosion's mind off the race.

Gary continued his call. "No change in position. Rio is still alive, for now, on the outside. Supreme Explosion is at the rail, but badly lathered and now a bit foul-gaited. Half in a blistering 52.3 seconds."

Then Vatter screamed as loud as he could. "SUPREME EXPLOSION OFF STRIDE, SUPREME EXPLOSION OFF STRIDE, AND INSIDE THE PYLONS. SZ flips Blue Man a left-handed Zander salute. She hits the lights and sends Rio forward. Hyphenated is second but struggling to keep up. I can't believe what the hell I am seeing. Fired Up Rio is flying down the backside opening up distance with each stride. Being parked for the torrid first half hasn't taken its toll. She commands now by three, make it four, no make it six lengths. She reaches the ¾ pole in 1:19.3! No trotter has ever gone that fast. Third quarter was 27 flat. Stephanie Z is chilly in the bike as they approach the head of the stretch."

I had a good view with the binoculars, and I saw what I hoped I wouldn't see. Rio was swishing her tail. Stephanie tried to ignore it, and Rio took a bad step.

Gabe went crazy. "Rio foul gaited. Stephanie takes the whip to her."

Stephanie whipped. Rio went faster and still swished her tail. Stephanie kept at it. I knew she would get fined, even during Millions Week. She was flailing at Rio's ass something awful as they hit the top of the lane. I knew Stephanie didn't want to do it, but Rio left her no other option. That big filly wouldn't be laying down to sleep tonight.

I was caught in a sea of pediatric humanity. They were rolling their arms in a backwards circle, like a third base coach sending the runner home. Vatter described the stretch run.

"The Army is demanding more. Stephanie asks Rio for more. Guess what? She's getting more and more and more. This monster filly is flying down the stretch. On your feet folks, this is history in the making! Fired Up Rio by ten and driving to the wire. She wins by an amazing fourteen lengths. Check the board, mile in 1:46! No trotter has ever gone that fast! Now here comes the rest of the field in mid-stretch. Flying on the outside is Playful Platypus, blowing by the pack for second. Supreme Explosion recovers enough to finish a distant third."

I heard Azzie's voice. "Fire up the drones."

I looked at Joe. "Drones?"

"You know Azzie, the show girl. Just watch."

Stephanie did not turn Rio at the paddock to get back to the winner's circle. She stood up in the sulky and continued around the track waving to the crowd. That was much to the delight of the 12,000 plus fans saluting her from the rail. They must have bet Rio. The ones that bet Supreme Explosion were vomiting in the restroom or jumping from bridges. I hoped that Deuce and Knuckles took the bridge.

By the time we got everyone set in the winner's circle I knew what the drones were for. In the sky behind Rio they had written '1:46!' in the bright pink color that was the trademark of Exquisite Evolutions. Rio and Stephanie had set a world record for trotters of all ages and sexes.

372

CHAPTER 72

Fired Up Farms
2300 August 23

As best as we could figure we had almost $8 million coming our way. More than enough to pay off the creditors and give us a little breathing room. But Azzie pointed out that unless we found a solid revenue stream the school would be out of business by the end of the year. That was something to worry about another day. Tonight was about two things, celebrating and justice. Celebrating our win and delivering some justice to the cheating bastards who had been using PEDS.

At exactly 2 AM, Father Jonathan accessed the CIC registration website. It was down for maintenance as we had hoped. He clicked on the logo and immediately typed GENNY. He was in. I read the numbers as he typed. He then removed their corresponding "recognized as" numbers. Unfortunately, this was very time-consuming. To be safe he exited the system at 2:14. We had only "fixed" 12 numbers. The Supremes had raced 22 horses during Millions Week alone.

The group was up and still basking in the sweet sunshine of The Millions Week victories. Father Jonathan reported our success and explained that he felt confident we could finish the rest of the horses tomorrow night. Azzie reported that she and Dan had engineered the leaks about the athletes. The information was set to arrive in carefully chosen hands on Monday. That only left the "favors owed" group. Joe came up with a brilliant plan for those lowlifes.

I was up early and got to the Sunday paper before anyone else. There was a great picture of the winner's circle with Rio on the front page of the sports section. She, of course, looked awesome. I was so happy, then I got sad. It seemed like Rio and I were the only ones there without a partner. Mom was hugging Dad. Joe was goosing Azzie. PC had found a way to get his arms around Stephanie. Billie was kissing Jenny (That was new!) The bishop and Father Jonathan were dancing with a bunch of kids, and I stood there with my finger up my ass. OK, it wasn't up my ass, but I was alone.

PC insisted on a celebration brunch at the country club Sunday. Since he was footing the bill, we obliged. The whole gang was there. We ate and drank to our hearts' content. Dad even got a little pie-eyed. I stopped at the track to check the horses. They were all fine. I topped off their water and headed home for a rare event, an afternoon nap.

I must have been more tired than I realized. That nap wasn't interrupted until I woke to the alarm at 1 AM. Father and I finished our work at 2:15 and hit the hay. We finished "fixing" the numbers for the horses that the Supremes had raced during Millions Week.

CHAPTER 73

Fired Up Farms
August 25

I had set my television to wake me at 5 AM so I could catch the news. When it came on, I heard that Deuce and Knuckles had been arrested last night and charged with various crimes. I turned up the volume as the info babe covered more of the details. The on-screen graphics said something to the effect that justice had been quickly meted out.

She continued. "One of the swiftest deliverances of justice occurred last night in New Jersey. Thomas Hofecker II and Kris "Knuckles" Markovich were arrested, tried, found guilty, and executed last night. Their lawyers appealed the whole way to the Supreme Court but to no avail. Here is the tape of the execution of Thomas Hofecker."

There I was standing with the governor. Deuce was strapped to the electric chair. He had on an orange bowtie to match his jumpsuit. The governor turned to me.

"Dr. Zander, this man attempted to have you killed, tried to ruin your family and your medical career, and referred to members of the Always Hope School using the 'R'(etard) word. How would like him cooked?"

"Well done sir."

Deuce requested a final statement. It was permitted.

Deuce was choked up. "I sincerely apologize for the trouble I have caused. I deserve this sentence. Had I patterned my life and behavior to mimic the exemplary life of Dr. Zander, I would not have gotten this far."

That's the damn trouble with dreams. They usually start out a little bizarre and just when they get good someone does or says something that wakes you up. I was fine until Deuce made that statement. No level of coma would allow me to believe that. I was now wide awake. I turned on the television for real and was disappointed to hear no news related to the scumbags. But I clearly heard Dad calling me.

"ZZ, get your ass moving. We've got a lot to get done."

I threw on some clothes and found him in the kitchen.

"Do we really have to replace that pipe today?" I asked in the best whiny voice I could muster.

"Yes, we do. They are calling for a big rain tonight and I am worried that part of the track will get washed out. Ever since Mr. Morrison passed on, I have been ignoring a lot of routine maintenance on the track."

"That's the guy next door that had the quarry with his brother?"

"Yeah. When we bought the farm, they were so helpful. I mean, we were only here a week and they offered to build us a training track. They practically forced us. And you know what a gem this track is. Top of the line work and they wouldn't take a thin dime."

I thought I had the answer. "Were they race fans?"

"Not exactly. I think they just wanted something to do. They had closed the quarry and I think they were bored. Their youngest brother just passed away and they said they needed something to keep them busy. Some project to take their mind off their grief. They started the morning after his funeral. After that they came over every now and again to watch me train, but they seemed more interested in keeping the track up to snuff. They touched up the surface and banked the turns twice a year. Took them 10-14 days each time."

I was impressed. "Nice guys!"

"Yes, they were. When Gene, the older brother died, he left $250,000 for the school. They were very helpful when we built the school. They handled all the excavation and grading. Of course, for no pay."

"Where is Frank? Wasn't that the younger brother's name?"

Dad responded. "I don't know for sure now. I heard he got Alzheimer's and was in a nursing home. He had no close relatives, but some distant related scumbags sold the quarry to Deuce supposedly to get the money to take care of him. Instead, they took the money and dumped Frank in a VA Nursing home. I visited him once, but he had no idea who I was. The home was deplorable, so I never went back."

We brought the backhoe over and set it up in the infield. Stephanie wandered over and wanted to operate the backhoe, but Dad had other plans for her.

"C'mon Stephanie, you know we are shipping out five with Tim Dempster this morning. Help me out by getting their tack together and assisting Timmy.

"OK Dad."

Dad was relieved when Stephanie left. "Whew, that was close. The last time I let her run that thing she knocked down an electrical wire, and nearly electrocuted me. Then she ran over the bench I made for your mom, near her flower garden. She may be a whiz with horses, but she can't operate a backhoe worth a shit."

I laughed my ass off. I wasn't talking to Dad at the time that incident occurred, but I remember Stephanie telling me about it. Somehow, she told a different version. I suspected that Dad's story was closer to the truth.

"ZZ, you can take up the first 18 inches quickly, but we will have to dig the next six inches by hand. Frank Morrison made a big deal about the 'magic tarp,' as he called it. He told me that the track base was large-diameter sandstone. On top of that came smaller diameter sandstone. That was covered with a very expensive tarp that was about 24 inches from the surface. He said that the tarp protected the base from water and ice damage. They put limestone on top of the tarp, with a large diameter at the bottom and the diameters getting smaller closer to the surface. The top was a fine dust. For some reason, he was always most interested in keeping the tarp in place."

"How are we going to do that when we have to replace the pipe?Didn't you say that the pipe was 30 inches down?"

"Yep, we will dig the last six inches of limestone with a shovel to carefully expose the tarp. Then, we will cut it cleanly with razor knives. You get to suture it back together when we are done."

"I can do that." At least it won't need any anesthesia.

The first 18 inches was easy as the backhoe did the work. The next six inches was a little tedious. However, an hour after we started, we were brooming off the tarp. I made the cut down the middle and rolled the tarp up to each side of the trench. I started to dig to expose the pipe as Dad watched. When I threw my third shovelful out of the hole, he interrupted me.

"Hold it. What is that at the bottom of the hole?"

"This?" I asked as I threw it to him.

He examined it for a minute, then he screamed, "I'll be damned!"

He ran into the house and I followed him.

CHAPTER 74

Fired Up Farms
0600 August 26

I woke up at 6 AM Tuesday and tuned into Marie Bartriromo on Fox Business. She was in a complete tizzy about something. Then I saw the graphic.

"Competition Integrity Committee computer hacked and controlled by NJ hospital operators and harness horse magnates."

I turned up the volume and hoped this wasn't another dream.

"Thomas Hofecker II was arrested at his home in New Jersey last night. He was charged with income tax evasion, conspiracy to fix gambling contests, conspiracy to defraud the government and other charges to be determined. Also arrested was Kris Markovich, a long-time friend and business partner. They raced harness horses under the name Supreme Stables and owned a for-profit hospital in Krenshaw, New Jersey named Supreme Medical Center.

"The FBI received an anonymous tip that the pair had the ability to deceive the CIC system into reporting negative results for grossly positive tests. The alleged perpetrators are accused of selling on the black market what they called 'get out of jail free cards.' For a fee, they would guarantee that their clients would not have any positive tests coming out of CIC. CIC was the only lab permitted by law to do such testing for sports teams and horseracing interests.

"Fox Business has also learned that every horse that raced for Supreme Stables in the past two weeks tested positive for performance-enhancing drugs, or PEDs, for short. The CIC is fully cooperating with investigating authorities. The FBI and Florida Department of Law Enforcement Criminal Investigations Department are now working together on the investigation.

"The governors of New Jersey and Florida have taken possession of all split samples kept at the CIC for the past six months. They and their police agencies will oversee the security of those samples from now until official testing by the CIC. An attempt to take immediate possession of the split samples by the FBI was blocked by the governors.

"According to affidavits more than 200 professional, college, and Olympic athletes are suspected of having purchased 'get of out jail free cards' from Hofecker and Markovich.

"The names of those involved will not be released until all confirmatory testing is performed. It is anticipated that this will be completed by Friday. The agencies have promised that the names of all individuals testing positive will be released.

"A deep confidential source has told Fox Business that known PEDs-laden samples were tested against every person identified and that they all tested negative.

"The FBI and FDLE would not confirm nor deny that report but did indicate that they planned to test split samples on file for all individuals identified as soon as this week. The original samples for all individuals had tested negative.

"We reached out to the six professional sports leagues identified, and to this point, we have received no comments. The NCAA has refused to comment until they gather further information. The International Olympic Committee would not speak with us. We were able to reach The United States Trotting Association. They, at least, have promised a statement before noon. Stay tuned for further details as they become available."

I heard Father Jonathan let out a primal scream. I ran down to the kitchen where Mom and Dad had been sitting and watching Maria. We hugged and looked up in time to see Stephanie slide down the banister while flipping double birds. She executed a perfect landing at the bottom of the steps. She bowed to the applauding crowd and proclaimed. "I am so happy I could just fart." We all nervously waited. Nothing happened. Stephanie smiled and said, "But I won't."

CHAPTER 75

Fired Up Farms
1900 October 6

I assembled the group to share the results of the research that Jenny and I had done. We gathered in the living room with popcorn and adult beverages. I began my explanation but was stopped after the first sentence.

"So, all of this was about gold?" Dad asked. He had a confused look on his face.

"Yeah, Dad." I replied. "Jenny and I think we figured out most of what went down, but the details are fuzzy. To our best guess, the story went something like this:

Dr. Hofecker was doing a medical school rotation at the VA hospital in Brockton."

"Isn't he the guy who lost his dick?" Dad interrupted again.

"I heard they reattached it, but it's the same guy." I sipped my beer. Before I could resume the story, Stephanie raised her hand.

"Yes Stephanie."

"Will it work? I mean, can he?"

I was losing my patience. "I have no idea, why don't you call and ask him?"

Mom chided me. "Zachary, be nice to your sister. But other than his reproductive system, how is he doing?

I was anxious to get to the story, but Mom never asked for much, so I obliged her.

"He has recovered from most of his injuries. He is in neuro-rehab for patients with traumatic brain injuries. I guess he can walk, but his speech is poor, and they are worried about his cognition. I heard it is unlikely that he will ever practice medicine."

Father Jonathan rose and led us in a prayer for Hofucker. I participated. I never liked the guy, but he had an uphill battle ahead. I prayed for him and wished him well.

I continued and hoped that I would get out more than one sentence before another interruption. This was a long story, and my bladder was already feeling the effects of two beers. Silence. I was pleased.

"When he was at the VA hospital, he helped an orthopedic surgeon relocate the shoulder of a veteran. The old guy had Alzheimer's disease and had fallen and dislocated his shoulder. When the procedure was done Dr. Hofecker was alone with the patient and a student nurse. He was to monitor the vet until he recovered from the sedation. We were lucky enough to find the student nurse and she told us the story.

"Dr. Hofecker was sadistic. He mocked most patients, and often played games with them to amuse himself. The veteran had been given some versed as a sedative, which got him talking gibberish. Dr. Hofecker decided to have some fun, so he asked the vet. 'What secrets would you like to tell me?' He figured the guy would say something about cheating on his wife or some other juicy tale. Well, the dude says. 'I got 20 tons of gold.' Dr. Hofecker just laughed and told the guy he had 20 tons of belly button lint. A few minutes later, the patient woke up and Dr. Hofecker went his merry way. The nurse told us that she and Dr. Hofecker concluded that no one with twenty tons of anything would be stuck in that VA home. It was substandard.

We got lucky when we identified an old army buddy of Deuce's who was still in the service. In light of the heat on Deuce he didn't mind telling us everything he knew about him. Somehow, he may have gotten the mistaken impression that Jenny and I were from some government agency."

Jenny interrupted. "I have no idea how that could have occurred."

Everyone laughed. I got back to the story.

"Deuce and he got together for dinner. After a few drinks, Deuce told him he wanted to hear the story about the Iraqi gold. Our contact felt that it was an old wives' tale. But Deuce wanted to hear the tale.

The gold was taken by the CIA from one of Saddam Hussein's many hiding places. Supposedly there were 20 tons of pure gold. The gold arrived at an Air Force Base in New Jersey. The plan was to send the gold to Nevada to be unmined."

Joe was baffled. "Unmined?"

Our contact had explained that to Jenny and I. "Supposedly the CIA was going to find an abandoned gold mine in Nevada. They would then buy it under the pretense of using it for special ops training. The real purpose was to crush up the gold and mix it with ore from the mine. They would then pretend that they found gold in this abandoned mine. The CIA would sell the gold and keep the money. They could of course never admit that they stole it. This was their way of 'laundering' the stolen gold and picking up secret 'off the books' funding for their clandestine operations.

"But according to the story, the gold was stolen during transport from New Jersey to Nevada. The truck and the soldiers supposedly escorting it were eventually found at the bottom of a river in the truck. The soldiers had been shot to death. Their murders have never been solved.

"There were no traces of gold in the back. But the truck was in the river for over a year, so that may account for no traces being found. People have been poking around Jersey looking for that gold for years. Some people think there never was any gold. Others think it is somewhere between New Jersey and Nevada. Still others swear it is somewhere in Jersey.

"Deuce also shared with his friend some information that his friend did not know. Deuce had learned through his own research that the government suspected that three brothers named Morrison were somehow involved."

Dad leapt from his seat. "You couldn't mean the Morrison brothers who owned the quarry?"

I shook my head. "The very same ones. Dad, you knew Gene and Frank. They also had a brother Harry. Harry died a few days after the date the army truck disappeared. Harry had a lengthy criminal record of felony burglaries. Frank was a metallurgist who did contract work for the government. He specialized in gold, of all things. Brother Gene operated the quarry next to our farm.

"Deuce learned that Frank had been a prime suspect. It was rumored that he had been hired by the government to oversee the 'unmining of the gold.' But he had five solid alibis that he was in Nevada the entire week of the alleged gold burglary. Harry died before he could be questioned, and Gene denied everything. He claimed to be at home or working the quarry the entire time."

Jenny and I kind of had to guess at the next part. "Frank returned home for Harry's funeral. After that, he approached Dad about building a training track. Dad, I remember you commenting many times about how insistent they were, and how quickly they built it. Do you remember how long it took them?"

Dad thought for a minute. "Six weeks or less."

I nodded. "That fits the timeline. During that time, he and his brother crushed the stolen gold and mixed it with sandstone. That mixture made up the deep base of the track. The "magic tarp" they put down was meant to demarcate the location of the gold-containing rocks below it."

Dad interrupted. "Come to think of it, they were excessively fussy about the deep base. Frank said something like 'it all rests on that.' If I recall, they used a number of men and equipment to excavate the track oval. But when it came to adding the base and the 'magic tarp' only Gene and Frank performed the work. Once they applied the tarp the original crew of workers finished the job."

Jenny jumped in. "If I was hiding dead bodies and twenty tons of gold under a tarp, I might call it magic too!"

I continued the tale. "Two months after the robbery the government thoroughly searched the quarry and came up empty. Gene and Frank's attorney cooperated until after the search was completed. When that came up negative, he threatened to go to the media with the story if the government persisted investigating them. That's when the government walked away from the case.

Twice a year, under the pretense of banking and renewing the track, they dug up a section. They took some gold and stone mixture to the quarry. Frank worked his metallurgy magic to make gold trinkets and small bars that they sold in the Far East and India. Most of the money they got they lost in Atlantic City. One was into blackjack and the other into craps. They were famous at the Borgata. They practically built the place.

"This went on until brother Gene died in a car wreck. Frank was never the same. He went downhill fast. He ended up in the hospital and then the nursing home. He only had a few distant relatives. They eagerly, with Deuce's help, got control of the property and sold it to Deuce. He tore the place apart and found no gold. But Deuce never gave up. He caught a break at the time he was selling off the equipment that the old guys had left over from the quarry. Knuckles, of all people, decided to test some of the stones he found in the rock crusher. Lo and behold, there were traces of gold!!

"It didn't take too long for them to figure out that the Morrisons crunched up the gold and limestone to 'unmine' the gold like they had planned in Nevada. Eventually Deuce figured out that the gold had to be in our training track. He tried to buy the farm but you refused to sell. Around this time, Deuce and Knuckles hit the jackpot with the CIC scams. They were making money hand over fist at the track, and with the athletes. Not to mention betting.

"But Deuce had to have that gold. He also had a thing for Always Hope. He felt she would be the trotting broodmare of all time. He had contacts in the venture capital business and knew that they lost their shirts when Justin McGregor died. Deuce and Knuckles located a very unscrupulous attorney who convinced the investors to go after the endowment for The Always Hope School.

"They were able to cripple the endowment, but you and Mom still would not sell. That prompted Deuce and Knuckles to arrange Ken's death. They did not want you dead because of the insurance policy you had. But they had to get you out of the picture. So, you had to live and go to prison. They were hoping I did not come back. When I did, they first tried to ruin my medical credentials. They parlayed that ruse into a suspension of my harness licenses. When it looked like that might fail, they forced Jenny to attempt to kill me. Sick bastards. All they wanted was to get the farm and Always Hope.

Epilogue

Fired Up Farms
0800 October 26

By sheer coincidence the Dying Was Easy gang was the first to arrive for the group meeting. Joe and Azzie grabbed a comfortable couch. Father Jonathan staked out a lounge chair that he barely fit into. I joined them and pulled up a small chair.

Joe began the discussion. "I can't believe that there are no sports to watch this weekend. ZZ, are you racing anywhere? I must have something to watch, and I am not a big fan of NASCAR or golf."

Father Jonathan laughed. "You caused some of this problem. I have to commend the sports leagues for the actions they have taken."

I concurred. "Taking a three-month pause was appropriate. I hear they are using the time to interrogate everyone involved. They have vowed that any owner, trainer, or agent that encouraged the use of, or made available, PEDs or 'get out jail free cards' would never work in the professional sports world again. I got the feeling they meant it."

Azzie added. "I also congratulate them for realizing that most of their athletes did not cheat. I know there were calls to cancel entire seasons, and to skip the Olympics for four more years. That would have been unfair to those who played by the rules. Resuming seasons and Olympics after a three-month investigation is appropriate."

I added. "I also agree with a one-year suspension for any athlete involved. They don't deserve a life ban like the guilty owners, trainers, and agents do. But they sure need some punishment."

Azzie recalled an area of unfinished business. "What about the 'favors owed' people. Those scumbags merit some ill to befall them."

Father Jonathan giggled. "The letters went out today."

I jumped up. "What letters?"

Father continued. "The ones that identify them as having been done favors by Deuce. The letters advise them that if they voluntarily go to the authorities, admit their guilt, and accept all consequences, their stories will remain confidential."

Azzie was surprised. "Who arranged those deals?"

Father laughed. "No one. There are no deals. Joe and I are hoping these goofs are dumb enough to turn themselves in. We made it all up. Can't you see it now? They show up at various police agencies pleading guilty to crimes that no one knows anything about. In some instances, evidence might exist to allow them to be charged. But in most cases, they will just make asses out of themselves and confuse the authorities."

Azzie grinned as she asked. "Most of the favors were blood alcohols that Jenny switched. Buster, for example, killed that lady in the crosswalk because he was drunk. Couldn't they have Jenny testify that she switched the tubes?"

I answered. "Sure, but since she threw the original tubes out, there would be no actual evidence to convict anyone of DUI."

Joe spoke up. "But if Buster or that bitch Bradshaw inadvertently say anything incriminating when they confess, the police might be able to do something. You never know. It's probably the best we can do."

Father topped him. "That's a good start. Wait until a month from now when the leaked story comes out. It will name names, dates, and dirty deeds that were covered up. These socialites hate nothing more than being exposed. Justice will be served.

Azzie was concerned. "What about the ones that come clean, as the letter advises? Don't they deserve a little mercy?"

Father Jonathan disagreed. "Tell them to look it up in the dictionary. Sorry for their luck. We are naming everyone."

0900

There were smiles all around as the rest of the participants arrived.

Dan took roll call.

Dan Santucci (present)

Zachary Zander (present)

Carl Zander (present)

Mrs. Zander (present)

Stephanie Zander (present)

Joe Crinelli (present)

Azquela Huggins (present)

Father Jonathan Young (present)

Johnson Stevens (present)

Jenny Rich (present)

Dan stood and began the meeting. "All present and accounted for. Before we begin today's business, I have to ask each of you a question under oath. Father, please use your Bible to swear everyone in after I swear you in."

After we were all sworn Dan asked a group question. "Since the date and time that Carl and ZZ discovered the gold in the track have you told anyone outside this room about the finding? If you remember, I made it clear to all of you the need to keep that information close to the vest. Please take a minute and be sure. An incorrect answer, even if accidental, can mean dire consequences for us all."

Each member of the group answered "NO" when called upon.

Dan recorded the answers. He looked relieved as he continued. "Today, we will review what we have learned to date and present a summary of the financial picture of the school and farm. I am pleased to inform each one of you that we have been extremely fortunate to have secured permanent funding for the school."

Dan's presentation was interrupted by loud clapping and cheering. Dan smiled and raised his hands to quiet us. He then continued.

"I will review in detail, later this morning, the confidentiality agreements that I had to sign to insure the deal. You each will have your own. Briefly, after today, there will be no further discussion by any member here of any discovery of gold at the farm. That never happened. It was a fictional end to the rumors that circulated around New Jersey for years. Any breach of our agreement will result in severe consequences for all of us. Not just the person or persons who improperly disclosed information. In addition, any breach will permanently end all financial support for the school. Each of you has worked hard and risked your lives for the school. Please, after today, forget everything you are about to hear."

Dan took a sip of coffee and then continued. "We sent the gold nugget that Carl and ZZ found for analysis. We had hoped to retain an expert to evaluate the source and determine the likelihood that further gold existed. Prior to that occurring I was contacted by an emissary from the Treasury Department. A deal was reached. No admission was made, but I think it is safe to assume that our gold was the gold that was taken from Saddam Hussein by the CIA. Obviously there is significant interest on the government's part to keep that a secret.

On the table, there is a jackpot lottery ticket and ten instant scratch-off lottery tickets. Those tickets are ours. The instant lottery tickets came from the six professional sports leagues. They want to show their appreciation for cleaning up their sports. The jackpot ticket is for the benefit of the school. Those tickets become ours when we sign the confidentiality agreements".

I objected. "Dan, why in the hell would we take a chance on a few lottery tickets when we had a megafortune in gold? Why do we give a shit what the government wants? And big whoop, we save professional sports, and we get ten scratch-off tickets? Cheap bastards. Dan, I can't believe you think this is a good deal for us."

Dan shook his head and grinned. "I knew I would get those questions. I can't believe you beat Azzie or Joe to the punch. I would have guessed that they would have been the first ones in my face."

I was embarrassed. "Dan, I'm sorry. I should have let you finish."

Dan walked over and patted me on the back. "ZZ, it's that fire, and spirit, and the courage to take anyone on that makes you tick. Please do me a favor and never change. But you are right. There is more. First, if it becomes public that the USA took the gold from Iraq there will be those who demand that we give it back. We would get nothing. Second, if it was reported that gold was discovered on the farm the whole state of New Jersey could be dug up by speculators. Third, if we put our gold up for sale in one block, we likely would tank the price of gold. All of those are bad for us and feared by the government. So, here's the deal: Each of those instant lottery tickets is a million-dollar winner from ten different states. We each get one to cash. After taxes, that should leave each of us with around $600,000."

There were gasps in the room but no one spoke.

"The jackpot ticket is the winner of $934,000,000."

No gasps after this bombshell. I had to look around the room to be sure people were breathing. Mouths were open but nothing was coming out. Dan refocused the group.

"The gold that never existed was worth $850,000,000. Due to the 'unusual' nature of the find only a very expensive clandestine firm could be trusted to handle the extraction and sale. Their cut was $150,000,000. That left $700 million for the school. The sports franchises, Olympics and NCAA added $234 million, and that's how the $934 million was the final total. I propose that Azzie claim that ticket. She will then donate the entire proceeds to the school. Since the school is a non-profit, there will be no taxes. With Azzie's current wealth, no one will question the massive donation. She will reap great PR benefits for herself and her companies as her compensation.

"The annuity will pay over $56 million a year for 30 years guaranteed. After that time the principal of $934,000,000 can be reinvested. The school will be financially set forever!."

Cheers and screams erupted. Cheeks were covered with tears. Dan again focused the group. "Now, I love you all, but I don't want to live with you for the rest of our lives."

Everyone looked confused.

Dan grinned. "As I mentioned, there is a penalty if anyone divulges anything they weren't supposed to. I have helped to create evidence that incriminates all of us in a conspiracy to fix the lottery in which the school won $934 million. There is also evidence in existence that each of us figured out a way to obtain our million-dollar tickets by nefarious means. If anyone discloses anything they shouldn't, the school will lose all of the money, and we will go to federal prison for a long time. We don't have to accept this deal. But if we don't, I can pretty much guarantee that we will be battling with the government instead of benefiting from their generosity."

Azzie raised her hand. "Do we have to take the million-dollar ticket? I personally don't need it. I would just as soon donate it directly to the school."

Jenny and PC joined Azzie. Neither one thought they should accept anything, and that all proceeds should go to the school.

I spoke for the Zander family. "We cannot accept any money. With the funding for the school secured we are solid financially. We made enough this summer to pay off all mortgages on the farm. Our racing stock is top in the country. Most importantly our family is back together. We don't need the money."

Dan shook his head. "I appreciate everyone's generosity. But we each must cash our ticket. We each have to claim the winnings and pay our taxes. Acceptance of the money implicates us in the fraud charges they will use against us if anyone talks. The government was insistent that everyone here agree to these terms. The terms are not negotiable."

Dad slowly rose to his feet. "Can we somehow get a share for Celeste Harrow and her son? After all, they lost Ken. And the insurance company clawed back their settlement once it was proven that the accident was staged. I know they are suing Deuce and Knuckles but so is everyone else in New Jersey. They don't stand to get much if anything.

PC spoke before Dan could answer. "It seems as if we each have to claim our tickets and pay our taxes. But there is nothing to stop us from gifting a portion of our after-tax earnings to a fund for Celeste and Carl Harrow.''

Dan and PC babbled back and forth about how the fund should be legally established. After they finished their ''shop talk'' we voted unanimously to each gift $10,000 a year to the fund from our personal accounts.

In the end, we all signed. I scratched my lottery ticket, and guess what? I won $1 million. Magically, so did everyone else. There would never be another word spoken about any supposed gold found at the farm. The company responsible for the total renovation of the track indicated that we could be training over it again by Thanksgiving. We had a lot to be thankful for.

ACKNOWLEDGEMENTS

Completion of this book marked a milestone in my life. Milestones are not often reached without help. I had plenty of encouragement and assistance to get me to the finish line.

It started with my family who tolerated me blabbering endlessly about the book. The folks at Dorrance Publishing educated me about the publishing process and guided the release of the original edition, *Dying Was Easy.*

Friends and family voiced their enjoyment and approval of the book. Although I appreciated that, what where they going to say? "Larry, your book sucked?" So, although their comments were important to me, I needed further unbiased validation.

I thank the many folks who shared online reviews of the book. I was humbled and encouraged by their ratings and kind words. So much so that I endeavored to improve the work and seek marketing expertise. Hence the revised edition.

A shout out goes to Kayleigh Fontana and Kate Rock for their assistance in publicizing this revised work. Kudos to Panda Publishing for their professional guidance in getting it edited and formatted.

Special thanks to one of my best friends from high school, Andy Muffley. Andy recently retired as an English teacher. He was kind enough to proofread *Dying Was Easy* after it had been published and to offer suggestions for its improvement. I am glad he didn't grade it. I tend to get a little sloppy with trivial things like sentence structure, commas etc. Andy doesn't. He marked up the whole book! Of course he was right. The book is better, and I am a better writer for his efforts. Someday I may pass his course.

ABOUT THE AUTHOR

Larry Kachik, MD grew up in western Pennsylvania. He obtained his premedical education at The Johns Hopkins University and received his MD degree from Jefferson Medical College. After finishing his residency, he began his career in emergency medicine. His clinical work in the emergency department spanned twenty-five years and included fifteen years as the Chair of his department. In addition, Dr Kachik also was appointed as the medical director of an acute care hospital.

Upon completion of his clinical career Dr. Kachik transitioned to working as a physician surveyor for The Joint Commission. He surveyed acute care hospitals, critical access hospitals, Department of Defense hospitals and hospitals run by the Bureau of Prisons. He also participated frequently in "for cause" surveys done to investigate serious hospital complaints.

Dr Kachik became infatuated with harness racing while in college. Shortly after he began to practice medicine, he embarked upon racehorse ownership. Over a span of greater than twenty years, he owned interests in more than fifty harness horses. He is still an avid race fan to this day.

www.ingramcontent.com/pod-product-compliance
Lightning Source LLC
Chambersburg PA
CBHW062112290726
48975CB00001B/205